The Longest Goodbye

Endorsements

"LOSING A PARENT IS ONE of life's most difficult moments and, in some cases, a difficult season. Shelly's heartwarming, poignant, personal account of her decade-long journey of saying goodbye to her mom who suffers from memory loss will be a source of comfort and hope to anyone going through a similar experience."

Carey Nieuwhof

Bestselling Author, Speaker, and Host of the *Carey Nieuwhof Leadership* Podcast

"IN *THE LONGEST GOODBYE*, SHELLY gives us hope and help to navigate when a loved one faces memory loss. Shelly shares her decade-long journey watching her mother decline with Alzheimer's disease. Through heartfelt stories and reflections, she gives her readers a glimpse into the pain of seeing a loved one slowly fade away while at the same time looking for hope-filled moments along the way. Shelly expresses how joy and pain can co-exist and where to look when everything feels lost. And most of all, her experience shows how the bonds of family and unconditional love carried her through. This book isn't about the clinical part of the disease; it's about the heart and how to hold on through all the seasons of memory loss."

Kevin Scott

Author, Leadership Expert, and Co-founder of ADDO

"IT'S MUCH EASIER TO WRITE fiction than to share a hard, human story of love and loss for others to read. Shelly has brilliantly authored pages that share the hard and the good of loving someone fiercely, while losing them slowly to Alzheimer's. Shelly is both honest and honoring with her words as she draws the reader into the journey of the one thing she feared most—her mother's diagnosis and slow decline due to Alzheimer's. Shelly's words paint a stunning picture of a brave and tender response to human suffering. Be moved in the reading of this beautiful remembrance."

Cathie Ostapchuk

Author of *Brave Women, Bold Moves*

Co-Founder and Lead Catalyst for Gather Women

Host of *The Strong Way* Podcast

"IN *THE LONGEST GOODBYE,* SHELLY invites her readers into the journey of her mother's battle with Alzheimer's disease. From the strong bonds of their special mother and daughter friendship to becoming a stranger to the mother who cannot remember, Shelly writes with the honesty and insight of a daughter processing the frozen grief of Alzheimer's and the long thawing of emotion, awaiting death's second chill. If you or someone you know is dealing with the pain of losing someone before they are gone, this book is a companion on your journey. Written as a friend who understands and with the wisdom of a faith holding on to hope, this book is for you."

Matt Tapley

Lead Pastor, Lakemount Worship Centre

"SHELLY LEADS HER READERS THROUGH the stages of saying goodbye to someone who is still physically present as they live with dementia. Woven throughout the book are firsthand stories of how her family wrestled through the realization that life was going to look different and how God met them in the joy and in the pain. Shelly beautifully describes her deep assurance she is still known, seen, and loved by her mom. What a gift this journey will be to so many others as they navigate Alzheimer's disease with their loved ones. Shelly's words will be comforting, relatable, and hope-giving to others walking this same road."

Melissa McEachern

Chief Operating and Content Officer at Crossroads Christian Communications

A FAMILY'S HOPE-FILLED
JOURNEY THROUGH ALZHEIMER'S

The Longest Goodbye

SHELLY CALCAGNO

AMBASSADOR INTERNATIONAL
GREENVILLE, SOUTH CAROLINA & BELFAST, NORTHERN IRELAND
www.ambassador-international.com

The Longest Goodbye

A Family's Hope-Filled Journey Through Alzheimer's
©2022 by Shelly Calcagno
All rights reserved

Hardcover ISBN: 978-1-64960-469-9
Paperback ISBN: 978-1-64960-203-9
eISBN: 978-1-64960-337-1
Library of Congress Control Number: 2022945171

Cover Design by Hannah Linder Designs
Interior Typesetting by Dentelle Design
Edited by Katie Cruice Smith

Scripture taken from the Holy Bible, New International Version®, NIV® Copyright ©1973, 1978, 1984, 2011 by Biblica, Inc.® Used by permission. All rights reserved worldwide.

References made to the show *This Is Us*, Created by Dan Fogelman, Los Angeles: 20th Century Fox, 2016-2022.

AMBASSADOR INTERNATIONAL
Emerald House
411 University Ridge, Suite B14
Greenville, SC 29601
United States
www.ambassador-international.com

AMBASSADOR BOOKS
The Mount
2 Woodstock Link
Belfast, BT6 8DD
Northern Ireland, United Kingdom
www.ambassadormedia.co.uk

The colophon is a trademark of Ambassador, a Christian publishing company.

Mom,

I never wanted to write a book about losing you.

I didn't want to say a long goodbye.

But I'm grateful for all these moments and all your love.

Table of Contents

Foreword

I WASN'T PREPARED FOR HER to go. To have her sit right beside me yet be so far away. It's been the longest goodbye. And I keep asking this question—how do we love through the hardest of days? Through the pain and the loss? Listening to the slow ticking of the clock as we sit watching everything slip away? There's no easy answer to my questions, and I've come to realize that we do the best that we can. We look for glimmers of hope, reach for deep grace, and collect all the precious memories and moments into a big pile of legacy love. We treasure each goodbye like it's the most important moment we've ever had.

Because it is.

CHAPTER 1

Yellow Flowers

I REMEMBER WHEN I FIRST learned about Alzheimer's disease. My parents moved to Ontario when I was three years old, leaving their home and families back in Newfoundland. Because of the distance, we didn't see our grandparents and extended family often. But I remember all the times we visited; they are written into my heart as some of my favorite childhood memories. Running up my grandma's hill that overlooked the bay, her freshly-baked bread toasting on the stovetop, my beloved cousins who lived down the lane, the china jug and washbasin in the room where I slept with the cupboards in the wall, family jigs, and getting into trouble for picking all the strawberries from the garden with my cousin. Many memories, considering the distance between us all.

But the one trip that stands out in my mind as I think of those days is the visit after my grandfather was diagnosed with Alzheimer's. I remember being a little apprehensive as we prepared for our trip, being a young girl and not really understanding fully what he was going through and what to expect. But our mom assured us it would be okay. It just meant Poppy was forgetful, but we didn't need to be afraid, so we bravely went with open hearts to see her family again.

Most of the visit, he sat quietly, and he didn't really know we were there. He was always a gentle, sweet man, yet I wasn't sure how to act around him in this new stage. I remember my mom being sad and having conversations with her sisters, as they tried to figure things out and work on a plan to support my grandma. I'm sure it was hard for my mom, living so far away and coming back to see her father in his declining state and not being part of the day-to-day care as his illness progressed.

I have one vivid memory when I think of that trip. After I became more comfortable and felt less fearful, I would often sit beside him—he in silence and me trying to be close and present. I remember I was wearing a blue sweatshirt and my black Adidas track pants in all my awkward, preteen glory. We sat quietly that day as I leaned up against him, across from the cuckoo clock in the room with the red carpet and all the family pictures and treasured dolls—in the house where my mom was raised. And out of nowhere, he said my name.

"Shelly."

The joy that spread through me was instant. I remember running to my mom and grandma and saying, "He knows who I am."

I wasn't forgotten, and that filled me with joy. In that moment, he was who I always knew him to be, and I was his granddaughter who had traveled far to visit. And he remembered me.

That was the last time I saw him, the last visit we made before he further declined. I remember when he died and how hard it was for my mom; yet in the middle of our grief, we never could have imagined what was still to come.

A few years later, my mom's brother was diagnosed with Alzheimer's—another gentle and beautiful soul. They had always been close throughout their lives. I remember him bringing me chocolate bars and playing classic Newfoundland songs during our visits. He loved music and had an instrument I'd never seen called a zitter, and I would sit and listen to him play it for hours. He brought life and light to each room he entered. I would feel so loved when I saw him, and I would get so excited when we would drive across the island and make the stop to see him and his family. Then, I learned he wasn't well. That was devastating for my mom; she loved him so much. She took his passing hard, especially after losing her father to the same disease. I can remember her sobbing, her heart broken at another loss.

But that wasn't the end.

Her oldest brother was diagnosed next—another one of my favorites with his big, loving personality and sparkling eyes. I would always be so thrilled to see him, too, when we would visit. I'd wait at my grandma's house in her little mudroom, almost holding my breath until he would burst through the door to see us shortly after we'd arrived. He'd laugh, give me a big hug, and call me the special nickname he had used for me since I was a little girl. The patriarch of the family. The brother they all looked up to. Unfortunately, Alzheimer's had become part of his story, too.

The last time I saw him—maybe a year before he passed away—he held my hand, and we walked together around the bay in the little Newfoundland town where he had lived his whole life. I can still feel his hand in mine. In many ways, his memory was going, but he knew every detail of everything we passed and told me all his stories. Those are precious memories stored in my heart forever.

When he passed away, my mom didn't get a chance to grieve him properly. I know she would have; she loved him dearly, too. But she couldn't remember him. Or me. Or anyone anymore. My sweet mom has Alzheimer's, too.

The fourth one in her family. It's enough to break your heart—the unfairness of it all that one family would have to bear such heartache. And now I sit beside her in the small room at my parent's house that has been her world for the last couple of years. Miles and miles away from her Newfoundland home and the longest goodbye journeys that happened in her absence. She missed the passing of her older brother, then her mother, and a thousand other moments and memories that happened in her presence that she never even knew.

I call it the longest goodbye—this losing of the one you love. Piece by piece. Stage by stage. Hour by hour. So slow, yet so fast that it all doesn't seem possible when you look back and realize that it's been almost ten years.

And now, she sits in silence on her chair, with pretty, rose-colored pillows surrounding her. I hold her hand; and I say her name; and I help her walk. I stay so that my dad can go and breathe and have some space. I sit by someone I don't know anymore, but whom I've known forever. All my life is wrapped up in her, and she's here. But she's also gone. And she's still my mom.

Sometimes, I think back, and I wonder if she was aware of what was happening to her. She was a nurse. She must have noticed she was forgetting things. She knew it was a chance, given her family history. I remember the first time my brother wondered if something was wrong. We were at my parents' cottage, and it was spring. Dandelions were sprouting up across the lawn, and she was trying to talk about them. She couldn't remember what they were, so she called them yellow flowers, and my brother noticed. And he had a thought that maybe it was happening to her, too.

Yellow flowers. That's when life started to fall apart.

For me, it was the combination of a few things. My mom loved Christmas, and buying gifts for everyone was always one of her favorite things to do. Each year, we'd plan a Christmas shopping day. We'd have lunch at our favorite steak sandwich spot and then spend the afternoon together tackling her Christmas list. This was one of our special yearly traditions. The fall after yellow flowers, we set up our shopping day and met at the mall. It didn't take long for me to notice that things weren't right. I was helping her get gifts for my nephews, and she couldn't remember what she had already bought for them. We wandered around the toy section for an hour, and no matter how I tried to help, she just didn't know what she needed to get. Then, I noticed when she went to pay for something, she would hesitate and was unsure of the pin code for her bank card; I had to help her. Then, I saw her struggle to pull the correct money from her wallet. I had knots in my stomach and felt like I was going to be sick each time we were paying for something in a store. I knew deep down that something was wrong.

The biggest thing I remember happening that day was when she had no idea where she had parked her car. Not a clue. I had seen her arrive, so I knew the general area, but we literally had to walk up and down all the rows pressing the key alarm trying to figure out where her car was. I was relieved when we finally found it but concerned as she left to drive home, hoping she knew the way and praying she would be okay on the roads.

It wasn't our usual Christmas shopping spree. After that day, I was full of continuous stress and worry. I knew what was happening, even if I couldn't say it out loud.

Then, I started to see it more. When she made my favorite coffee cake, it didn't turn out because she missed some ingredients. When she came to babysit my children, she wasn't sure where their school was. I had to unwrap Christmas gifts she had already wrapped because she didn't know what was inside. Then I had to read her cards to her after her seventieth birthday party. When she went to Florida, she bought me three of the same kind of my favorite perfume. And I noticed she would ask me the same question a couple times.

We had moved on from yellow flowers.

I was in denial for a long time. I couldn't talk about it; I didn't know how to bring it up with my dad. I was afraid to have a conversation with my brothers. My beloved aunt came to visit from Newfoundland, and I didn't even see her while she was here. I knew she would know that her sister was different, and I didn't know how to process what was happening with words.

I read the book *Feeding My Mother* by Jann Arden that year, in preparation for what was ahead. It's a beautiful book, filled with endearing stories and lovely recipes; and while I loved the words and sentiment, it further scared me and made me want to curl up and hide away. I read it again a couple years later, and it felt different. I could see things more clearly, but at the time, I had to put it away on the back of the bookshelf and forget the words I had read. I needed to pretend that wouldn't be my story or my mom's story. Even though I knew it would be.

Avoidance was easier on my heart—on all our hearts—for a long time. I feel a peace now that she didn't know what was happening, that God allowed that grace to her, because the thought that she did know and didn't want to tell us or talk about it is just too much for me to bear. That's a hard path to navigate alone. But maybe the slowness of the longest goodbye for her was so gradual that she didn't know she was slipping away. That's what I choose to believe because that's what I saw, and that's what my heart needs. It was painful for us, but it was seamless for her.

And now we sit together. I put her feet up. I play her music, switching between comforting hymns from the Gaither Vocal Band to the sentimental Newfoundland music of Shanneyganock. We watch a million Hallmark movies together and all the *Little House on the Prairie* episodes that we loved when I was a little girl. Most of the time, her eyes are closed, but she's not asleep. I know she feels my presence. It's been months since she's said my name and looked at me like I'm her girl. But I know I am. I am hers, and she has always been mine. And nothing can take that away. Her memories may be gone; but mine will live on, and she will live on through them.

It's spring right now, as I write this chapter. And outside the window of my office, our front lawn is filled with yellow flowers. Every year—and likely forever when I see them—I'll think of the year when we first realized that our mom was beginning to slip away. It's ironic that those yellow flowers eventually turn white, and then they just wisp off in the wind. They slowly let go, and they fade away in a gentle farewell as they trickle across the sky.

Yellow flowers blowing in the wind. Saying goodbye.

Reflection:

When you or someone you love begins a journey of illness, it's normal to take time to process. Change is hard. Relationships are complicated. Grief is real. Take the time you need to sort out your feelings and emotions. If you don't know what the path ahead looks like, it's okay. You will get there. Be patient with yourself in the process.

CHAPTER 2

FOR MANY YEARS, I WORKED as a pastor, looking after the spiritual needs of children and families. I was a young mom, and my husband and I worked together at our church to best meet the needs around us.

There was a young girl named Sarah who would come to our children's program on the church bus. During the week, she didn't have a ride to our building, so we would get in our van and drive across town to pick her up—with our toddler and baby in tow. We tried to support her and her mom. She was a sweet and kind girl. And I think she loved feeling like part of our family.

Time passed, and we moved away and eventually lost touch. But years later, I ended up working at that same church again. One day, just a few weeks after I had re-joined the staff, a call came in from a mom who wanted someone to come and pray for her daughter, who was dying of cancer. I couldn't believe it. It was Sarah. In their darkest hours, her mom remembered the love shown to their family by the church. And she remembered me.

So, I went to Sarah. I sat by her bed, re-united with this adult whom I had loved as a child.

She looked at me, and the first thing she said was, "Why?"

I told her I didn't know; I don't always understand life either.

She told me she was scared, so I held her hand. In my shaky voice, I shared with her the Source of my hope. How my faith had seen me through many storms. I reminded her of her own faith that she'd had when she was a child and how that faith was still real and available to her. I shared how the unconditional love that had rescued me could still rescue her. She nodded when I asked if she still knew Jesus and all the love offered to her. I sat beside her bed and looked at the bright childhood posters she still had hanging on her wall of kittens, puppies, and sparkly stars; and my eyes filled with tears as I thought about full circles, deep pain, planted seeds, and love in broken-up places.

I went back a couple days later, and she couldn't talk anymore. I sat by her bed and read to her from my Bible. A few days later, we got a call from her mom saying she had passed. She was at peace. Heart settled. Her pain gone. And I'm full of thanks that I got to sit beside her, grateful that I entered her life again, even if just for a short time. And I believe *that was perfect grace.*

Since then, I've often thought of the simple question she asked me. The first thing she whispered as she lay there in her pain after all those years of not seeing me was, "Why?" And isn't that the question we all ask in the middle of it all? When pain is right smack in our face and the hard things of life are closing in? I know I've whispered it in the dark loneliness of night when everything is too much to bear, after the fountains of tears have been shed and my heart can only offer up a faint beat from its dry and parched place. Why?

We see those we love slipping away. We are helpless and full of pain. Bad reports, sudden loss, often side-swiped by the unexpected. Life is not always what we planned or hoped. Sometimes, it's tempting to stand on a mountaintop and scream out *why* to the world. Some days, the heart is just so full of things that hurt. There is no perfect life, no matter how much we wish we didn't have to experience pain.

I remember after my brothers and I noticed things were changing with my mom and we acknowledged it to each other. Our conversations were like soft whispers we would share between ourselves. We didn't really want to talk about it, but we knew it was necessary. I couldn't talk without becoming overcome with emotion. I didn't want to be weepy and upset, but I couldn't process the pain.

Eventually, we determined that we had to talk to my dad about what was happening. For some reason, this was the hardest thing in the world to do. It's one thing to wonder and talk with your siblings, but for us to have to bring it up to our dad just seemed like too much to bear. Having him agree would be the worst thing. It would mean it was really happening.

So, we planned it out. One day at the family cottage—my mom's favorite place—the four of us stood together on the front step. The grandkids played by the river with Grandma—as they always did—not at all aware of what was happening or what would come in the years to follow. She pushed them on the old rope swing, their laughter and joy echoing across the water.

We asked our dad if he had noticed any changes and told him that we were concerned with what we were seeing for ourselves. It was gentle and kind; it was painful and heart-wrenching. We loved our parents so much, and our mom was our life. How could this be happening? I don't remember all that was said. But he knew it, too, even if it was a reluctant acknowledgment. I remember hugging him at the end of the conversation and seeing he had a few tears, something that I'd never observed from my strong father. And I remember thinking at the time, *Why?* Why our beautiful mom? Why our family? Why do we have to go through this? Why?

Those were painful days. But in the middle of it all, there was one thing that I held onto with all that I had. My mom loved a lot of things. She loved her husband and kids, her grandkids, her friends, her church, shopping, a cup of tea, decorating, cooking, gardening, and the list goes on. But what I knew without a doubt is that Mom loved Jesus most of all. And the Jesus she loved so much is the Jesus Who has given His peace to me in the middle of all my *whys*.

There were more hard conversations to come. A heartbreaking meeting at the Alzheimer's Society with a case worker that none of us were ready for. Sharing with my children about what was happening with Grandma. Conversations with her family and friends. My brave brother even visiting to ask my darling mom if she had noticed any changes in herself. Days of deep pain, often with my stomach in knots and my heart in my throat.

The question *why* makes up a big part of life. From a sweet girl lying in bed about to breathe her last breath to a mom forgetting a life filled with so much love. *Why* is hard. I don't know why Sarah had to die of cancer in that bed. I don't know why my mom had to be the next in her family to get Alzheimer's. I don't know why I've had to sit by and watch her fade away over the past ten years when I feel like we still had so much living to do together.

I'll never really understand. I've accepted it's just part of life—for all of us. We all could share our stories that start with hard questions. But in the *why*, there has always been so much love. Thankfully, I haven't had to look too far to find those places of comfort. And then? A never-ending peace that runs down and overflows and mixes with grace. In the middle of all my *whys*.

Reflection:

Hard conversations take courage and bravery. Most of us want to avoid them at all costs because it's easier to pretend that everything is okay. If you struggle, you are not alone. Approach difficult conversations with love and grace. If it's hard for you, then you can be sure others are struggling, too. And most of all, it's okay to ask why. Sometimes, life doesn't seem fair; situations feel too difficult to comprehend; and pain is real. Wade through the grief; let yourself feel what you need to feel. Why is never the wrong word to think or say.

CHAPTER 3

Find Your Bricks

THE LANE THAT LEADS FROM the blue Newfoundland house on the hill down to the water's edge in the little town of Dildo (yes, the town made famous by Jimmy Kimmel) is probably one of my favorite places. I love that path. It's hugged by wildflowers and a wooden fence, and I'll forever be captivated by the old homes still standing that belonged to my mother's family in past generations. Most of the houses are deserted and empty now, barely holding on as the rickety walls work together to stay standing.

One of my English professors once told me that I had a sense of history because I always wonder what happened in the past in places about which I knew nothing. I'd stare up at glowing high-rise windows driving through a strange city and think about all the people inside, living lives that I knew nothing about, all connected to generations and people before them and after them. Or I'd be fascinated by old, historical places that hosted stories from the past—centuries before I stood on those same grounds in my worn-out tennis shoes sipping my coffee from the Tim Horton's drive-thru, still being able to feel a sense of the history all around me.

Those houses on my grandma's lane bring out that "sense of history" strong in me. I go deep into my daydreams and wish I knew all the stories those walls contained. If I wasn't positive there were giant bugs and mice inside and that the walls wouldn't collapse on me, I'd love to go in and look around. I'd think about what happened to make the families walk away and wonder why part of their past stands there abandoned and alone, boarded up on the lane down to the bay.

The last time I got to visit those houses on the lane, I was on a special adventure with my mom. Each year, she would take a trip in September and go back to Newfoundland to see her family around my grandma's birthday. She would normally go alone, but she couldn't travel anymore by herself as she was becoming more confused. So, my dad would go, but he had decided that the last time they went together would be their last trip. I think it had become too hard for him.

But now, there we were. Her and I.

It all happened because of a friend at work. At the time, I was co-hosting segments on television, and I was getting my make-up done by Anna, a beautiful and creative soul with whom I loved to talk. It's especially easy to chat with a make-up artist when she's making you pretty, painting away all your insecurities and seeing your vulnerabilities. Over time, I had shared with her about my mom and our journey. I remember telling her that my mom wouldn't be going to Newfoundland that year for the first time in many years and that I was sad she would miss her trip and that she wouldn't likely be able to go again.

Out of the blue, Anna said five words to me, "You should go with her."

I hadn't even considered it really. I think the idea scared me a little. My mom was still high-functioning at that point; she could still communicate fairly well and take care of herself, for the most part. But she had definitely declined and needed extra care, and I just wasn't sure my heart could handle it all.

I remember saying to Anna, "I can't; it will be too hard."

And she said again, "You should go."

So that night, I called my dad and asked him if I could take Mom on her yearly trip. He was surprised, but he said yes. I think it was a break for him, too; and when I look back, that week was the last time he fully had time to himself before he really dove into being a full-time caregiver.

So, the plans were put into place for our trip. We called my aunts, and they were so excited that we were coming—both of us together. My grandmother was in long-term care, and I knew she didn't have much time left. I was so thankful I would get to see her, too. It had been twelve years since I had last visited. Life with a young family and all that entails had made my trips less and less frequent.

My grandma still owned her beautiful, blue house on the hill at the top of my favorite lane. Because we were coming to visit ("coming home," as they say), my mom's sisters decided they would open up the house, and we would all stay there together. It really was the most special thing that they could have done, and I still tear up when I think about what a beautiful gift it was.

My mom and I got through our flight together without any issues, and soon, we were back on "the rock." I remember my uncle picking us up at the airport and driving to the little town. I held my breath as he turned and began driving up the familiar road from my childhood. And there it was, the beautiful, blue house on the hill, waiting to welcome us. And while I know houses aren't alive, I felt as we stepped inside that it wrapped us in warmth, love, and memories of all the days that were lived and loved inside those walls, of which we had been a part. Especially my mom.

The trip was a glorious mix of pain and beauty because don't those things often just flow together? My mother was in the stage of knowing-but-not-knowing. She was so happy to see her family but couldn't really express it. She knew everything was familiar but couldn't quite communicate what she was feeling. She would know us, and then she'd forget. But despite it all, she was content, and the familiarity of her home and family made her happy.

I will treasure that trip for the rest of my life. Watching my mom do her make-up in the morning. Helping her choose her clothes for the day. Tucking her in at night. Sharing a bed together in my grandparents' old room, where I remember snuggling up to my grandma when I was a child. Hearing her breathe beside me. My heart breaking and filling all at once.

We made the most of every moment—looking over the ocean from the cliffs of Brigus, walking the sands at the breathtaking Salmon Cove, and taking pictures as we marveled over the colorful sheds in Cavendish. I sat on a cod-gutting table that looked out to the sea, went on an adventure with my uncle to a hidden pond on a quad, and let the joy of those moments and all the memories from the past fill my heart. We laughed, went through photo albums, made fried-dough toutans, danced to Newfie tunes, and walked down around the bay holding hands. I can close my eyes now and feel the love of that week. The embrace of family and love. The covering of home, bringing comfort.

And then, we went to see my grandma. My greatest fear was that she (then in her nineties) might not know me. Another reason I was afraid to get on that plane. It had been so long. Much had changed.

We drove to the beautiful home that was caring for her. We walked down the hall toward her room, and I could feel my heart beating out of my chest. My heart, that I often tuck so deep to protect it from things that might bring pain, felt as vulnerable as it ever had. But I chose to be brave. I had traveled far. This is also why I came.

My aunts went in first and got my grandma ready for our visit. She was having a good day. And as I went and sat by her bedside in her new home that I had never known, I began to cry. I remembered all the childhood visits with my brothers and my parents, the smell of her fresh bread, her cozy hugs, the joy when she came to my wedding, the pride when I brought my own children to meet her. So many memories as I sat and looked at her dear face.

My aunt leaned over to her ear and whispered, "Mom, remember that little baby? The one that Sheila and Byron chose and then brought to the house to meet you? Do you remember her? Shelly?"

That was the moment. My heart that has always longed for belonging with every beat stood still.

"Indeed, I do," she replied.

I felt my heart pulse again, those words bringing incredible life. She knew me. I was remembered. Loved. Accepted. Embraced. But also broken as I watched my own mom, standing by that bedside, too, not really knowing her own mother. And that shattered my heart. Because as much as I loved my mom, I knew she loved hers, too.

The longest goodbye hurts in so many ways.

My heart was filled in countless ways over the next few days. I spent time feeding Grandma blueberries, and we brought her apricot squares that she had bought for me from the bakery on my last visit. I sat with my mom by the bedside of her mom, visited with cousins at a big gathering back at my grandma's house, went for walks and had heart-to-heart talks with family, and felt like I was with those who understood the path and the pain. Most importantly, I watched and learned from those around me who had already been on this journey how to love and care through all the stages of life. Good and bad. Joy and pain. Happiness and deep aches. What I call the "glorious mess" of life. All the things I was living and that I knew would get harder and harder.

The day before we left, I walked down my favorite path on the lane, past the abandoned houses, and then to the creaky steps down to the dock that had been in my family for generations. I sat and looked out over the water into the bay, as I ate my packed lunch in quiet and let myself be filled with the beauty around me, processing all that was happening in my heart. I started to explore as I walked further down to the beach and climbed over the rocks. Then I got a little brazen. I felt greedy asking for more. I knew the trip was gift enough. But I went ahead. I prayed a little prayer to my Maker. "Send me a treasure."

I didn't really know what I was looking for, but I asked anyway. I kept walking, and then I noticed something on the beach amidst all the stones, rocks, and sticks that had washed up on shore. It was an old brick. It seemed a little strange to find a brick on the beach. I took a closer look and picked it up. I couldn't believe my eyes. It was faded and hard to make out. But that brick had a word on it: *Smith*.

Maybe I read too much into things, but I had just asked for a treasure. I was on a trip that was all about family. And there in the sand was a beaten-up brick with the one common thread that ran through my whole journey—my mother's family name. Smith. What a precious gift.

I wrapped up that old brick in one of my sweaters and packed it in my suitcase to bring home, and that piece of weathered stone is now in my house. I can see it right now from where I write. From the beaches of Newfoundland to the vineyards of Niagara was a reminder that God hears me when I call, that I am known by Him, and that I have a treasure in legacy. It is a reminder of the gift in that trip with my mom and how my heart was mended by love, even when it hurt and was in shattered pieces. When it seemed I was losing everything, I still had so much.

A few months later, I made the journey to Newfoundland again for my grandma's funeral. I stood by her casket, looked at her beautiful face, and was grieved by her loss. I was so thankful I had gotten to say goodbye, that I had been given those moments with her. Then, I wept because my own mother wasn't there beside me; she hadn't made this trip with me. Her last trip home was the final one for her. She didn't know her mom had died, and she never got the chance to really say goodbye. It was all just a little too much for my heart to process. I felt so alone, responsible to carry her grief, too, because she didn't understand the loss. I know she would have felt it deeply.

After the funeral, I took another walk down my favorite lane before I left. I thought about my brick from the last trip and all that I had been given despite the losses. I went back up to my grandma's blue house, and my aunt and I cut off snippets of red winter berries that were decorating the hill that I loved as a child. I gently wrapped them up in a paper towel to be the treasures that I brought home this time in my suitcase. I placed the little branches of berries around my house and was reminded again that we can find gifts in hard seasons. When we get worn and beaten down, it's tempting to close off ourselves. It feels easier to let our hearts become like the boarded-up, empty houses on the lane and just walk away. But no matter the journey—no matter the cracks and imperfections and the effort it takes to keep standing—there is always hope. There are always gifts to be found.

I also gently took a rose from my grandmother's casket, and I brought it back home to my mom. A small reminder of the woman who loved her, even though they never got to say goodbye.

Reflection:

Keep looking for gifts on your journey. When days are hard, it can be easier to avoid things that hurt and to give up on moments of happiness. Don't let yourself shut down; it's often in those challenging and pain-filled moments when joy bursts through the darkness. You will never regret letting yourself feel and experience love. Look for the gifts that can be found, even in the hardest of days. Let the way that you embrace the hard things be part of your own story in the longest goodbye journey.

CHAPTER 4

All the Moments Matter

I REMEMBER WHEN WE WERE kids and my dad would pull out the slide projector to show us old pictures. (If you are under the age of forty, you can search "slide projector" in a search engine to understand what I'm talking about.) I'm fairly certain he still has it in his basement somewhere. We thought it was so cool when he placed the slides so carefully in the round tray and then set them on the machine. We'd all sit around together in the family room as he clicked through the snapshots.

Moments from the past. Click. Click.

Looking back over the last few years, I feel like I've been in one of those old slide reels. I haven't lived days as much as I've lived moments—the kind of moments that are seared onto my heart and have brought a change of perspective to my life. I could easily pick out dozens that are etched into my mind. Moments showing joy, laughter, family, pain, beauty, connections, surprises, grief, reflections, goodbyes—and the list goes on.

Click. Click.

We don't always value what happens in the little moments. Yet in the fast pace of life, moments are the key part of living. When we don't embrace them, they slip away. When we don't appreciate them, they pass us by. When we fail to recognize what happens in the small, we get lost in the big. Our moments matter.

Sitting in that dark room as a kid, watching and listening to the reel click, I remember saying, "Slow down, Dad! I didn't see that one! You're going too fast!"

I've always loved moments. And I've always been afraid to lose them. In 2014, a movie came out starring Julianne Moore called *Still Alice*. Based on the best-selling novel of the same name, the movie chronicled the journey of a linguistics professor diagnosed with Alzheimer's shortly after her fiftieth birthday. I remember when the movie was available to stream. There were so many times I would almost watch it and then change my mind and pick something else. I was terrified beyond belief to press play. It was still early in our journey, and I wasn't sure I could handle watching a story that we would likely live.

One night, when no one was home, I got brave and decided to give it a go in my dark room, bracing myself for what was ahead. It ended up being grueling for me emotionally, as I expected. I wasn't talking to anyone at that time to help process what I was going through; and like the Jann Arden book, I probably wasn't ready to consume an intense story that mirrored the one I was living. I lay in my bed when it was over, sobbing in the dark. I was in a daze emotionally for a couple weeks, wondering how we would ever be able to walk through what was coming. In hindsight, I know that was normal because no one is ever ready to deal with loss.

I do remember thinking as I watched the movie about how fast Alice's moments slipped away and how quickly she lost everything that made her who she was. It terrified me because I knew that would be our family one day, and I wasn't sure if we could handle it all. However, it also showed me how important it was to capture all that we could, while we could.

I also observed that despite Alice's memory loss, she was still the same person she always was and worthy of the love, dignity, and respect she had always experienced. She was changing, but who she was in everyone else's life hadn't changed. That spoke deeply to my heart and planted in me the resolve and importance of honoring and loving someone who is with you but slowly fading away. They still deserve all that they were worthy of before their diagnosis.

While mentally and physically, my mom isn't who she was anymore, she is still my mom. She will always be worthy of that place in my life, regardless of what her mental state is. Her role as my mother will never diminish or be set aside because of a disease. I made the choice early in this journey to keep honoring her as my mom, despite her limitations, and to celebrate the moments that mattered to her, even if she doesn't know they are happening. I refuse to let her fade away without any acknowledgment. I will respect her and love her, as I have done for my whole life. She is my mom. And all the moments that mattered before Alzheimer's still matter now. I've loved our moments together all my life. I've always treasured them. I didn't want to miss those moments then; I'm determined not to miss them now.

But it's not always easy. In the middle of our longest goodbye journey, I remember times that I've felt really overwhelmed. I'm the oldest child and an organizer of events, and I naturally love a good party. (I have a cupboard of supplies, and I can pull a celebration together in an hour if needed!) When my mom began to decline and couldn't do the things she had always done before for our extended family, I began to put all the pressure on myself. She loved a good celebration, too, and had so much fun making everything so special and wonderful for all of us. So, I decided I had to make things happen now. It had to be like it always was, and I couldn't let anyone down.

When I look back, I realize that the expectations I placed on myself were too much to carry on my own. I began to fail miserably. After a while, extended family gatherings started to become a time of extreme stress for me. I felt like I had to pull it all together, manage the family, handle the situation we were all facing, and make sure everything went off without a hitch. Then I'd feel guilty, and resentment would start to rise because I felt like it had suddenly become my responsibly to make everyone happy. Before a big family event, I would become an emotional mess, take it out on my own family, and dread what was ahead. It wasn't that I didn't want to be together. I just wanted everything to be the same, and I knew it wasn't. I couldn't manage how I was feeling. I felt angry, bitter, and sad; and I couldn't process my emotions in a healthy way.

Somewhere in that journey of despair, I decided that I couldn't make the world right again. It was too much of a load for me to carry. I decided that what mattered most to me was to be there for my mom and dad and let go of the rest. Maybe it was time to focus on moments, not mountains.

Christmas Day has always been a big deal for our family; my mom loved that season so much! For a couple of years, my dad and I tried to still make it all happen Mom's way. She couldn't help anymore like she used to, and for some reason, we thought we could be her. And boy, did we try! We definitely gave it a good effort! The father-daughter "pull off a turkey dinner like the ones mom did" seemed to be our goal, and it was a high one. (She was an amazing cook and made incredible meals!) But it wasn't the same, and the stress that I felt coming up to Christmas Day . . . Well, I don't think that's what Jesus had in mind when He wanted us to celebrate His birthday.

I would end Christmas Day utterly exhausted and defeated. It became a day where we were already struggling with the changes happening in our mom, and then we were reminded again of just how amazing she was at everything. And boy, did we miss her and all that she did for us. It almost made the whole situation worse because we saw again all we were losing. Our efforts came from the heart, but the stress to execute was just too much.

Finally, one year, someone had the idea to just order in food for our holiday celebration. The important thing was to be together. Why were we putting all this pressure on ourselves? That was one of the best decisions our family made. We adjusted, realized what mattered, and accepted that a new normal was okay. Who says you can't have take-out Italian food for Christmas dinner, anyway?

I think a thousand pounds of weight lifted off my shoulders. I didn't hate Christmas, anymore. I didn't have to pretend to be my mom, anymore. Things changed for me after that. I felt like there was permission to do things in a new way. I never stopped caring about everyone else, but I decided that when all was said and done, how I walked through this season was something I had to do well. I wanted to be able to look back and have no regrets. I couldn't be responsible for everyone else's journey or happiness, but I was in charge of my own. My legacy to my own family and how I loved my mom and dad in this season was the most important thing to me.

So, I stopped carrying all the weight, and I began to care more about the moments. I threw out the mountains of expectation. Moments are easier to handle, so I began to gather them up in little portions that I could manage and embrace. When I look back now, I have my own slide projector of memories of Mom during this longest goodbye season. And I can go as fast or as slow as I want to go through them. I'll have them forever in my heart; no one can take them away.

- Sitting on the couch together, hand in hand
- Going for a walk together around the neighborhood
- Making a trip to Tim Hortons and buying the muffin she wanted that she'd pointed out to me with a smile, then sitting by the fireplace in our favorite spot and enjoying our treats.
- Wandering through the pretty greenhouse looking at the flowers that she loved
- Sitting and listening to Newfie music that made her smile and tap her feet

- Baking at her house with my daughter at Christmas, while she wandered around and watched us, so happy we were there with her in her kitchen
- Walking around the cottage and sitting by the fire
- Holding her hand while watching the fireworks on the Grand River
- Flipping through the pictures in the photo box together in the living room, saying all the names of the people in each one
- Painting her fingernails on my back deck
- Watching her smile at her grandkids and hug them, even though she couldn't find her words
- Seeing her face light up at church when she would see me on Sunday
- Drinking tea on her back deck in Florida when my son and I went to visit
- Helping her up off her chair and walking arm-in-arm around the house
- Visiting every Wednesday and having dinner with her and my dad with my dad making her a little bowl of dessert after each meal because she loves sweets
- Washing and drying her hair in the kitchen and asking her if she liked it and her saying yes.

All the moments. They changed so quickly, so I try to make them and capture them all when I can. When it's too hard to fully comprehend or navigate the big mountain of what's happening, the moments bring it back to what matters.

Click. Click.

The pursuit of big and grand can't compare to authentic life lived in small moments. Small is what matters; big is overrated. All the things that I thought were important that I had to go after—none of those things compare to the precious moments I've captured with my mom—the moments that I decided were important, that I know she was worthy of, even if she didn't know they were happening. Each one will be valued, and the snapshot reel will grow. Pictures of life and love. Portraits of joy and even of pain. That's all part of living. The moments that we capture in our heart affect the choices we make as we go forward. What we value in our moments sets the tone for our living.

As I feel my mom's season fading more and more, I'm gently gathering up my precious moments more carefully. I've started to label them for safekeeping and listed them for future reference. I'll slide them one by one into my picture reel, so that I can pull them out whenever I need them again. I'm glad I was looking and listening. I'm so thankful I stopped to collect them and that they didn't pass me by. Just like that old family projector, I'll forever click through them one by one and slow down on the ones I want to remember. All our moments matter.

Reflection:

Don't look back with regret. All the moments matter, and while you can't be there for each one, make sure not to miss the ones that matter to you. Life will feel different on the longest goodbye journey; and some days, you won't know which way to go, so make the choices to embrace what you know matters. Adjust, refocus, and don't stop living or celebrating. Never underestimate the small, simple acts of love that you can give and receive as you are walking through a season of loss. There is much joy to be found in collecting moments. Moments allow you to write the joy-stories of love in hard seasons.

CHAPTER 5

My Mother and Mary Kay

ANYONE WHO KNOWS MY MOM is aware of how beautiful she has always been. I've known the same thing, too, for as long as I can remember. As a kid, I thought my mom was so pretty. As a teenager, I'd think to myself, "Wow! Mom always looks amazing!" As an adult, I wondered how my mom never seemed to age. She was just blessed with natural beauty and great genes. At times, I found it a lot to live up to—if I'm being honest. She just always looked so put together. She had great style, lovely hair, and perfect skin.

Speaking of skin, I remember when my mom first discovered Mary Kay cosmetics. This make-up and skin care routine that she committed to is a key memory from my later childhood years and on, and I'm sure one of her best beauty secrets.

As an awkward teenager, I was a little in awe of the Mary Kay legend and the stories about the pink Cadillac cars, the pink-clad women who ran the empire, and the miracle make-up so beautifully packaged in the signature hue. There was no social media for the first forty years or so of the company's existence—no Instagram reels with girls showing how amazing they look using the products or Facebook group requests to join online sales parties. (Please don't invite me to those.)

This make-up hustle grew its business through personal connection. Suburban communities, mom groups, and door-to-door salespeople spread the word about the incredible products that could transform your skin and life. It was one of the original multi-level marketing companies—right up there with Amway but for the bold, beautiful, confident woman who wanted to take on the world. My mom loved it all.

I remember when the boxes started coming to our house. She had found a Mary Kay make-up dealer (sounds so shady-glam), and she was hooked. Of course, the more you bought, the better the deals, and she loved a great deal. Much to my dad's chagrin, the boxes kept coming. The dealer's card was on our fridge; mom was a user, and Mary Kay was now a part of the family. I can remember her saying, "I need to call my Mary-Kay dealer. I'm getting low." There was no going back to the common drugstore cosmetic aisle now.

I also remember looking on wistfully from afar at her make-up and skin routine. With my terrible, adolescent skin issues, I was very intimidated by all the products that were now around the house. I secretly wondered if it would be the magic solution to my problems, but I didn't think my acne medication would mix well with expensive toners and moisturizers. I'd read the labels in secret and hoped that maybe one day, I'd have beautiful skin like my mom's and could enter the pretty, pink world of Mary Kay cosmetics. I wanted everyone to tell me how beautiful I was, too. I'd also need to find a good career because it wasn't cheap, as my dad would say whenever the newest order was placed.

I especially remember her nighttime routine and all the magical lotions—some for the eyes, others for the hands—the cleansing, the toning, and then the final step of pink emollient that made her whole face shine. And the smell? It was like pink heaven, a defining scent of our good-night hugs. I would say that for at least thirty years, Mary Kay was the first and the last part of my mom's day.

But now? It's probably been four years since my mom has done her skincare routine. The last time I can remember was when we were on our trip together to Newfoundland. Each day, I would sit on the edge of the bed and watch her put on her make-up in the morning and do her skincare steps at night. It was almost automatic for her, a learned process after so many years. Amid her deteriorating memory, she still wanted to look her best, and she remembered what to do. I thought it amazing that even as Alzheimer's was stealing her mind little by little, she still knew her skincare routine. No disease was going to take that away. Her Mary-Kay best always. I think it brought comfort to her, doing what she had always done. A rhythm of routine. She wasn't vain but always cared about how she looked and took care of herself. I found comfort in watching her do her make-up and clean her face like she always had done.

After that trip, things began to decline at a more rapid pace. It's often the pain of familiar things that hurt the most when you see someone you love slipping away. Over the course of a few months, I would go and visit my parents and look under the bathroom sink to see that her make-up was unused; and gradually, step-by-step, she stopped doing all the things she had done for years to care for herself. The lipsticks were becoming expired; the compacts collected dust; and the mascara had all but dried up. I knew it was just make-up, but it represented so much more.

One day, I went over, and I helped my dad go through some cupboards and clear out what she wasn't using anymore. We had decided that it was time. This is always a hard step in the longest goodbye journey. We did a good purge together, and after, he packed up a bunch of her Mary Kay products and put them by the front door for me to take. I always hesitate to take something of hers home; I usually cry for the whole drive. I'd rather life be normal and she still need it. But I took the bags he gave me—I wasn't kidding when I said she had a lot—and knew that she would have been happy to give them to me. I went home that night and got pulled into the pink, magical goodness. Even though the product was a few years old and expired (I rarely check the expiration dates on food either, and I'm still alive), I started using it. Mostly because it was my mom's. And I'd do anything to be more like her.

Before long, I was caught up in the world of Mary Kay, too—my teenage dreams of the pink skincare routine finally coming alive. I was especially intrigued by the thick, pink emollient, which I affectionately call face-shellac because I'm pretty sure it could literally hold a house together. It's my favorite product because it smells like memories of my mom, and I remember her putting it all over her face every night. I love to slap it on before bed each night, too, and it amazingly absorbs into my skin while I sleep. Now, I come home to my bathroom counter full of her pink skincare goodness. It seems strange that a multi-level marketing make-up line could conjure up such emotion and love, but whatever brings us comfort in our journeys and reminds us of the greatest moments of love in our lives is worth remembering.

Recently, I was at my weekly dinner at my parents' house. I looked at the side of the fridge, and I was strangely comforted that the make-up dealer's card is still in its place. I imagine it's been there for twenty years, at least. I'm sure when Mary Kay Ash started her make-up empire, she didn't know she'd be part of creating family moments or memories. Or maybe she did.

And perhaps, I'm a little odd for connecting my love for my mother to her skincare routine. Maybe it's weird to use her old, expired products. But I don't even care. I'll keep using it sparingly to make it last as long as I can. Beyond the make-up and skincare, I've decided it's okay to soak in whatever gives me comfort. We need to grab onto anything that gives us peace as we walk the journey of loss and helps us remember what was important to the ones we love. It's even okay to make those things important to us, too.

That's why I also keep a cute centerpiece in the middle of my kitchen table, planted bushes of pink roses in my garden, pick a fruit explosion muffin when I go to Tim Hortons, wear multiple Alix and Ani bracelets, and do a million other little things because of her.

I'll hold on to anything that wraps me up in the comforting reminder of all she has been in my life—pink expired make-up and all.

Reflection:

Whatever brings you comfort in your longest goodbye journey is okay. The items that remind you of the people you love are important and significant. Find whatever your "pink-packaged make-up" is. Look for those experiences, items, sights, sounds, textures, smells, and whatever else that connects you to the one you love and pull more of that into your life. Reminders of love in goodbye journeys bring comfort and peace.

CHAPTER 6

This Is Me

A COUPLE YEARS AGO, MY daughter and I got invested in the television show, *This Is Us*. Its beautiful and compelling storytelling—the narrative of a family—and their deep complexities immediately captivated me. I've spent many an episode sobbing over some of the storylines and depictions of family in the show. I feel like they have people on their writing team who have lived through some of the episode themes because the accuracy of the emotions that are expressed feel so real to me. Especially the ones I've experienced. (I could also need to go to therapy more, but that's beside the point.)

One of the storylines is about adoption, and as an adopted child, I don't think I've ever seen my own journey and experiences depicted in such a real and raw manner. The series is centered on triplets, one adopted, and their individual and collective experiences at all stages of life are central to the storyline. It follows the journey of their lives, the relationship between their parents, and the tragic loss of their father. It's made up of flashbacks and flash-forwards—some of the best storytelling I've ever watched.

I had finally gotten through the emotions of the adoption story in the series when that year's season finale showed a flash-forward of the life of the mom, Rebecca Pearson. I knew right away that they had set up her storyline to be that of a mom, wife, and grandmother with Alzheimer's. I sat there in tears thinking that I would have to quit watching the show. How is this so much like my life? Are they secretly following my journey and trying to mess with me? I was afraid it would be like the *Becoming Alice* movie experience, but now every week. I told my husband and daughter that was the end for me, that it would be too hard for me to watch. But I've held the course, and I've kept on going, unable to look away.

I know it's fiction, but there's something comforting about seeing your life mirrored in an accurate way—something about seeing that you're not alone and that others have walked through your life's journey and have struggled as well. It's a little strange that I've had to find that on a television show, but in an odd way, it's helped me feel normal. And also, at times, it's allowed me to cry it out, as I see the same emotions I feel but can't always express. Maybe it's also a good reminder that we do need to talk about these hard things more in life, to stop making the painful conversations off-limits, to make the emotions of real-life places accessible to others, so we don't feel alone. And while I have lots of support in my life, it's a little strange that I've had to find so much comfort in a television series.

And then, I go back to moms—Rebecca, the fictional one in my favorite television show, and my own, whom I see in her journey. There's just something about mothers, isn't there? I love my dad as much as my mom, but I would say that much of the loss we have felt in our family is because our mom was at the center of it all. Our guiding star. Our place of comfort. Our heart's home.

It's hard to lose her. So, I try to steady my heart as the beats change. There are a couple days each year that have always been hard for me, even before this journey—my birthday and Mother's Day. In the middle of my already-emotional life, the other component to my identity is being adopted.

The day I was born and placed for adoption and the day all about moms have always been complicated and complex for my emotions. That's probably why I always feel disappointed—nothing feels special enough, and I can't fully celebrate as I should. At times, I've been terrible to my own family, ungrateful for things done for me and unable to process or express why. I finally figured it out a couple years ago, so I know how to manage it better now that I understand the triggers. I've learned and walked through finding my identity, value, and worth. But I haven't always been my best self on those days in the past and genuinely didn't even know why. Then, I had to add to the mix my own mom fading away.

Raw. That's usually the state of my heart before Mother's Day now. It's probably the hardest day of all. It starts the week before, and the closer the day gets, the more my emotions rise. I remember a couple years ago, a few days before Mother's Day, I was visiting my mom, and she said my name. It was a beautiful gift to my heart. Then, that week, a picture of her popped up in my Facebook memories. She looked amazing, and my heart ached as I missed that version of her so much. I was happy she had said my name, but I felt angry for what I had already lost. On these special holidays, I feel guilty for wanting her back, even though we still have her. I was grateful the day she knew my name—that was a gift—but I wanted more. I miss my mom, even though I have her.

My heart misses our talks and the love she always poured into me. I want her to know all about my family and everything that's happening. I wish I had cherished the moments that I didn't realize were fading away. I feel like I would have soaked her in more and squeezed all the extra love I could from her.

Raw. Torn open. Wounds that are too hard to close. That's how the word *mom* makes me feel some days. Then, I think about mothering my own kids. How being their mom has been the greatest joy of my life. My own life-treasured relationships. Those whom I am hopefully loving and caring for with a mom-like heart. I think about those who hurt, those who wish for children, those who have lost children, those who can't see their children, those longing for a mom, those missing their mom, those who didn't have a good relationship with their mom. I think, too, about the mom I never knew, who gave me the mom I had. It's a long list of complicated mom feelings and circumstances for myself and, I know, many others.

A couple years ago, I went to see a therapist. I was trying to deal with all the loss I was facing. She encouraged me to find the things that give me life and make space for those moments. It was good advice because loss can make you feel empty. And when something is raw, you wrap it up so it can heal. So, I choose to be positive and feel love on purpose, especially where pain tries to take over. I reflect on all the gifts in my life and bandage myself up with all those memories. I try to remember what it means to mother, and I keep looking for ways in my own life to do it well.

I've learned to go to my mom on those hard days and cherish our moments even more. We walk around together. I help her eat, sit with her, bring her flowers and treats, watch Hallmark movies, and tell her she's the best mom in the world, even if she doesn't remember that she is.

One year, I wrote her this letter. She couldn't read it, but it helped my heart.

Dear Mama,

It's almost Mother's Day weekend, and this year, it feels harder than most. While I see you often, most days, you seem farther away.

I want to grab onto you and pull you back.

This walking loss is hard to comprehend, and I try to face it all with a brave heart; but sometimes, I'll find a quiet corner in a random parking lot and let everything out with a good cry. A few weeks ago, I was on Facebook and realized that I had years of past messages from you that I had never thought to go back to. I spent a long time reading through those messages, and it brought me so much comfort to see your words. To read that you loved me, that you were proud of me. To hear you talk about all the grandkids and our family. I could hear your voice saying you were praying for me. It was the most beautiful and the most painful two hours I'd spent in a long time. I read through all those messages and imagined we were talking in person. It was a cherished gift that made my heart both ache and fill with love all at once.

I love you, my mama.

I was thinking this week about what present I could get you for Mother's Day. I know you love flowers, and you always say they are so pretty, so I'll bring you a beautiful bouquet. Dad says you need some new pajamas (he's incredible and takes such good care of you), so I'll go get the prettiest ones I can find. I think of all the things that you love, and I want to surround you with what makes you happy.

As I was thinking about presents, I started thinking about presence. About the things that money can't buy. I thought about all you've given me over the years and how your presence has been one of the greatest gifts in my life.

I can look around our home and see the things that I do because they are things that you did. I always clean up the dishes right after dinner. Because you did. I have teabags in a little jar on the counter. Because you did. I have a weird Tupperware flour-shaker to make gravy that always makes a mess. Because you did. I hate crumbs on the counter, love hot drinks in a pretty cup, decorate for seasons, and make hello dollies every Christmas. Because you did.

Your presence in my life is strong. The woman that I am. The wife, mother, daughter, sister, friend, and everything else I try to be. I'm always wanting to be more like you. My faith and my passions. My longing to love other people well. All those parts of me have the fingerprints of your presence that have touched my life all these years. I want to be to others what you have always been to me. You've set a high bar, but I'll keep trying. And I think maybe now the best gift I can give back to you is presence, too.

So, I'll sit with you and hold your hand as often as I can. I won't leave. I'm right here with you, for all the days ahead. I love you, my momma. Happy Mother's Day.

Love, your girl

Life in general is complex. Families are complicated. Nothing comes easily or perfectly. But we hold on to things that we love, walk through seasons with grace, and manage the best we can.

I've learned to look for gifts in the middle of pain and mess because that's the only way I can move forward. That's how I look at the word *mom* now. And I often think that things wouldn't hurt so badly if I hadn't been loved so well, so that's another gift.

This Is Us, the award-winning television show that has eerily mirrored my life, is still on each week, and I faithfully tune in. I am always holding my breath as I watch a fictional family that has strangely brought me comfort and helped me process pain as they lose their mom, while I'm losing mine. It's been another helpful way to look at life, family, and journeys of love and loss.

This is my mom. This is our family. And in the middle of it all, this is me, holding on the best I can through all the days.

Reflection:

Holidays and special occasions can be so difficult as you walk through seasons of goodbye. We hold traditions dear, and when they change, we often don't know how to adjust to that reality. Allow yourself to feel, but gently make room for a new way moving forward. Remember that presence really is the greatest gift you can give or receive. It can feel painful, but try to embrace and fully love wherever you are in the journey. Hold on to the preciousness of the past while learning to navigate a new way ahead.

CHAPTER 7

When You Didn't Know It Was the Last Time

I THINK ABOUT "LAST TIMES" a lot. I can't help it. It's where I am in my journey. I remember something that my son asked me a couple years ago when we were on vacation. We were out walking, having one of our deep conversations (which is usually him talking and me listening), and he asked me something profound.

"Did you know the last time that you held me would be the last time?"

His words blew my mind and inspired me to try to pick him up on the path where we stood, so that I would, without a doubt, remember the last time that I held him. But he's over six feet tall; I'm not that strong; and I need my back for a few more years. I just stood there, a lump forming in my throat. I couldn't remember the last time I held him because I probably didn't realize it would be the final time I'd pull him up off the floor into my arms. He was growing and moving along in life. Holding just naturally transitioned to other expressions of care and affection.

Time goes by so fast—kids grow; mama's arms get smaller; and life never stops. We're always moving from stage to stage, living daily moments so fast that we never stop to think about the last times.

His question made me reflect then, and I still think about it now. I think of other moments that I never knew were ending—ones more painful than those of a little boy growing up too fast.

- The last time my mom would say my name
- The tearful kiss left on my grandma's cheek in the hospital
- The abrupt end of joy found in a job I adored
- The last conversation with a young friend at church
- The last visit to a place that deeply mattered to me
- The last time our family gathered at the cottage with both my parents
- The final time we'd all be together for Christmas dinner

I didn't know those were the lasts. What would I have done differently if I had known? What would I have said? Would I have ever been able to let go? Every day, we live moments that are important to us. We don't think about moments ending because we're too busy living in them.

There was another Sarah in our life, a precious girl whom we loved with all our hearts. Before I was married, I always dreamed and hoped that we would have another family in our lives who were friends but also family. Thankfully, we've been blessed by those relationships. But there is one extra-special family. We met in college, became friends, and did ministry life together on more than one occasion. And while the adult relationships were wonderful, what was extra-precious was the friendship between our kids.

My friend Lisa and I went through two of our pregnancies at the same time, and it was a joy to have a friend with whom to share those moments. Our five children combined were best friends, and some of my favorite moments and memories are the ones our families shared together—play days, watching each other's kids, birthday parties, swapping kids on Sunday mornings during ministry, beach meet-ups, family celebrations, and the list goes on. All our children were close (and still are).

But our two youngest, Hannah and Sarah, had a special bond. They looked like twins. Sweet and tiny, blonde girls who loved each other and chatted together like teenagers in their high-pitched, three-year-old toddler voices. Holding hands at church, bringing happy meals to their babysitter's house, dressing alike at the mall, growing up together making movies, playing, drawing, and buying each other BFF necklaces and t-shirts whenever they could.

Then, Sarah got sick with cancer. The beautiful girl, loved by so many, fought so bravely and loved Jesus with all her heart until the very end. I'll never forget picking up our kids early from school and telling them that Sarah had died. We held each other and cried over the immense loss that we felt. Then a few days later, I sat on Hannah's bed, and together, we wrote out the tender words to be shared at Sarah's celebration of life.

Standing at her graveside and holding our hands tightly as families and friends, we all tried to make sense of what had happened. We were broken-hearted and in shock that the girl we loved so much and was such a part of all our life memories was gone. My confused, young daughter made a memory box and filled it with all the sweet childhood pieces of their journey together. Bittersweet reminders of their friendship and love still sit on her closet shelf almost ten years later.

Most of all, I think about the last time we saw Sarah. Her family came over on a Friday night, like they had done a thousand times before. The girls got their dads to buy Kool-Aid to dye their hair. The older kids hung out in the basement and played together as they usually did. It was like all the nights we had ever been together, but somehow, it felt different just the same. Then, when the evening was over we said goodbye at the front door. We all hugged and prayed together and waved as they walked down our front steps.

That was the last time we saw Sarah. She went to her heavenly home not long after. I've thought about that night a million times; it brings tears to my eyes as I sit here and write about it right now. I wonder if we would have done anything differently if we had known it was the last time we would have all been together. I'm sure we would have hugged a little tighter and held on as long as we could. And those precious, little, blonde friends might not have been able to let go.

We didn't know. But I'm so glad we have that moment and all the others to fill our hearts.

Moments make our life—the good moments, the hard moments, the joy moments, the pain moments. We never know when it may be the last time for anything, really. So, we just keep living on purpose, with love and intentionality. Thinking about that affects the way I love my family, offer forgiveness, refuse to hold onto bitterness, and embrace whatever life brings my way. I don't want to forget or lose any seconds or regret what I didn't do. I want to look back on every tick-tock of the clock as part of beautiful stories written through faithful life-living. Even the moments I never saw coming and didn't know were ending—those are the moments when you know how real love is.

One day, I had my little boy up in my arms, and then I put him down on the floor and never picked him up again. It's okay that I never realized that was happening because I likely would have tried to hold on forever. One night, I hugged sweet Sarah at our front door, and it was the last squeeze I would ever give her. I would have hugged her longer if I had known and made sure she knew again how much we loved her.

On October 28, 2020, my mom looked at me and said my name for the last time, the final time she spoke to me like she had my whole life. If I had known, I would have never left her side. I would have begged her to call out again.

Every day, our moments change. Don't wish them away. Don't hold onto them too tightly. Make them matter because each moment is a gift. First and lasts. Beginnings and ends. Gather them into precious places; write them down in memory ink; and impress them onto your heart. Wrap your arms around them and pull them close. If it is the last time, you want to make sure you lived that time well.

Reflection:

Sometimes, moments are happening so fast that we can't keep up with them. Then, before long, they are gone, and we wish we had recorded them, valued them more, and held on tighter. Don't take your moments for granted. Record them; write them down; take pictures and gather all the precious seconds and minutes all around you. You never know when the last moments will be, so be a collector of all that matters to you, so you can look back with a heart full of love and no regrets.

CHAPTER 8

The Day I Found Out Who I Am

"WE WANT TO KNOW WHO we are." My son had gotten slightly obsessed with genealogy and our family tree. Being adopted, my biological background had always been a mystery to me and something my kids wanted to know more about. I could understand them being curious about the pieces of me that they carry. I had never seriously pursued finding my biological family. I figured I would look when I felt ready, even though I was curious. I also have an amazing family, and that was always enough for me. Usually on my birthday each year, I would spend some time looking around on some of the online search sites, just to see if anyone was looking for me.

There were never any listings for a baby girl born in Happy Valley, Newfoundland, on August sixth, so I would just go on with my life until the next year. But maybe, it was finally time. Perhaps I was ready to know more.

So, a couple months later, Mother's Day came, and I got a very unusual gift—a DNA kit from my kids. I promptly spit in the tube and sent it off. Either I would get answers, or I would be cloned by the government. I was willing to take the risk either way.

A few weeks later, I got an email with the results. I wasn't home but doing some work out of town, so I logged in to check things out. I sat there in a quiet coffee shop, and I felt everything around me disappear as I focused in on the report, learning things that I had never known before. It was like reading a secret manual about myself that had been hidden away. Some things were obvious. I'm more likely to drink caffeine than the normal person. I'm more likely to be sensitive to loud chewing. I'm more likely to be bitten by mosquitos. All of these DNA-supported facts were very true.

Then came the family tree information, which I had previously never known anything about. I'm British and Irish with a touch of Scandinavian (sadly, not a Russian princess as my son had hoped). I then clicked another link and dove into my health background—increased risk of celiac disease and diabetes. I sat there in Tim Hortons with my coffee with two creams and one sugar, hoping the cookie I just ate wasn't going to make me a diabetic while learning all about my DNA life, trembling a little as things unfolded before me.

Identity has been a deep struggle of my life, something that I have had to fight through in all my seasons. But as I sat there reading, I felt healing pour out on me as I learned things about myself that I had never known. I've been loved all my life, but in my deep places, there have been missing pieces that no one else could ever understand. Now I knew more about myself, and that was something I had always desired.

Then, I saw the connections button on my profile. I had read that sometimes DNA results could give you an idea of what your biological last name might be or where you had been born. I thought that might be interesting, so I clicked without giving it much thought.

One click. Then, everything changed forever. Immediately, I was looking at a list of hundreds of names of people related to me. At the top of the list were my closest relatives who had also done the test. An aunt and two cousins. I sat in that Tim Hortons and felt things start to spin. Another click connected me directly with my cousin. She received an alert that a new relative had popped up, and I was a close one. She messaged me almost instantly, and within an hour, I was learning about a life that I had been part of but never lived. I'd imagined it, but now it was real. The days that followed were a bit of a blur, as I tried to process what had been a question mark in my life since I was a little girl reading *The Adopted Family* book over and over each night with my mom until I wore out the pages. Everything had flipped upside down, and I was in a place I had never been. I was overwhelmed; I was terrified. I had answers; I had questions. I was grateful; I was alone. I felt connection; I felt deep grief.

In the middle of all this emotion, I learned that my birth mother had passed away. I hadn't decided if I wanted to meet her, but now I would never have the choice. In the middle of losing one mom, I found out the other one was gone, too.

I woke up one night gasping for breath, thinking I was having a heart attack. I went to the doctor the next day and asked for an ultrasound to make sure I wasn't about to die. A couple days later, I sat in my counselor's office crying so hard I couldn't breathe. She told me that adopted children have a legitimate and real connection to their DNA. What I had learned, what I was grieving, and what I didn't understand caused physical reactions that I had never before experienced. I sobbed, saying I had lost everything. All my moms were gone. I was an orphan now. She reminded me that my mom was still with me.

I walked around for a week in a complete fog, wondering how life could ever be the same, unsure of how to deal with all of this in a life already filled with things that were so heavy. There's much more to the story and still things to unfold, and I'm trusting God for the journey ahead, just like I do with everything else in my life. I do know that everything in our life has a purpose. No matter what we face, we can have peace; we can have trust—no matter the storm. *I am who He says I am*, I say to myself repeatedly. The plans for my life are good. I've been chosen. Loved. Cherished. Valued. I know these things; now I'll hold on tighter. *"You knit me together in my mother's womb . . . I am fearfully and wonderfully made . . . My frame was not hidden from you when I was made in the secret place . . . Your eyes saw my unformed body; all the days ordained for me were written in your book before one of them came to be* (Psalm 139:13-16).

A long time ago, there was a young teenager. I know her name now, and I know a little more of her story. I imagine she was likely scared, in a really hard situation. Without many options, she made a choice. She couldn't keep me, so she did what she felt was best. She is a stranger. She is my mom. She gave me life through a labor of love that was mixed with pain and heartache. I wouldn't be here without her, and my heart breaks sometimes when I think about her.

Then, there's another mom—the one whom I've loved since my earliest memory of us standing by the fence in our first backyard—the mom that I've always had. She came and took my little broken-up life and wrapped it up in pink, cozy blankets surrounded by cuddles and kisses. She surrounded me with love so tight and has whispered throughout my life that everything is going to be all right. She didn't give me life, but she is my life. She *is* my mom. I may have been given to her, but she definitely was given to me. I have faith because of her example. I serve because she did. I forgive because she was forgiving. I work hard because I saw her work hard. I love others because she loved with no end. I want to be like her in every way. The best mom in the world.

As I struggled to process who I really was after I found out about my birth family, I would sit close to my mom. Even though she couldn't talk to me in the way that I wished, I knew that she still felt my presence. Even though I had lost so many parts of her, in my own confusion, I would hug her, sit close, and hold her hand tight. I wanted her to know I was here, and I needed to know that she was still there, too. I would look straight into her eyes as far as I could, knowing that she could see how I felt deep into her heart. Our eyes said what our words couldn't, me still needing her so much in my pain.

"I love you," I say.

"You and me," she replies.

"Always" is my answer.

"You're so good," she says.

And my life is okay in spite of all the pain. I know who I am, and I know who she is. And now, I know where I started, too—another example of joy and pain, all wrapped up into the glorious mess of life. So, I offer up my thanks for it all.

Then I think about my first mother—the woman who gave birth to me, then placed me for adoption. I imagine her still being alive and going to meet her around the bay in the little Newfoundland town, not far from the one that I visited so often growing up, not even knowing she was close by. Her living her life, me living mine. Connected, yet strangers. I'd walk up to her front door; and she'd open it; and we'd look at each other in wonder and then slowly embrace. I'd imagine that we'd cry a little and wonder what life would have been like she had kept me. I'd tell her it's okay, too, and that I understand. I'd say, "Everything I have in my life is because of the choice you made. Thank you for giving me my family. Without them, I wouldn't be where I am today. I wouldn't have my faith, and I wouldn't be me. You made a choice that I'm sure was hard, and I will always be grateful."

Then I think about the mom who chose me. Every time I'm with her, my heart says, "I love you, my sweet mom. You are one of the greatest gifts in my life. Thank you for never letting go of me. Thank you for always cheering me on and believing in me. Thank you for praying for me when I didn't think I could get through the day. Thank you for loving your family in a way that makes me want to love mine, for being the mom to me that I've tried to be to my own children. There is no one like you. Your love has been a constant flow throughout my life. It rescued me, filling the deep places that no one could reach. Now, it's my turn. I'll love you forever, and I'm beside you no matter what is ahead."

I've had two moms, both wrapped in loss, both wrapped in love, both making me who I am. My life drastically changed the day that I spit into that

DNA test tube my kids gave me, but I'm glad I did. I'm glad I know who I am. I'm grateful for love that came from two different places.

Reflection:

Most of us experience times in life that come with pain and circumstances that we don't always understand. Our relationships can be complex, too, and we face hurt that can be hard to reconcile, especially when woven through other experiences in our lives. Be quick to forgive; don't hold on to the past. Trust in the Maker, Who has known all the steps of your life before they even came to be. Don't waste any moments holding on to grudges that will prevent you from saying the goodbyes that you need to say. Goodbye journeys are hard enough on their own, harder still when there's no peace present. Wrap up loss and grief tightly with love.

CHAPTER 9

Self-Care Soup

I REMEMBER FIRST HEARING ABOUT national Self-Care Day. I was in the middle of an emergency, and I thought that if anything was an illusion, then a day to take care of myself was certainly it.

There have been a couple of seasons with my mom when things went into crisis mode. I remember the first time, when we had to bring her to the hospital. My dad, my brother, and I took her. She was still mobile then and could walk and express herself still but wasn't understanding what was happening, and a change in environment was very jarring to her. Hospitals are not designed for people with memory loss or struggling with confusion. Getting her through triage, having to sit in a waiting room crowded with people, and the nightmare of getting bloodwork and then waiting to see the doctor almost pushed me over the edge. Never mind trying to get her back into the car after a long day of confusion. I feel anxious right now thinking about it. It may be the highest day of stress I'd ever experienced. And it wouldn't be the last.

There were other hospital visits and calls made to 911 that took up every ounce of emotional capacity that I had. Afterward, I would go home in a zombie-like state and literally lie in my bed for a day and not move. Telling my family that I needed to be alone, unable to even speak, I'd watch some mindless Netflix show and try to come down from the anxiety so that I could function again. I was also navigating a very stressful job at the time with high demands and no space to even recover before I had to go back to work. And that's just me. I can't imagine how my dad, the main caregiver, felt after those intense days, often bringing new challenges to work through and manage. Needless to say, I started to value self-care.

My therapist told me how important it is to find things, even little things, each day that are easy to do but help sooth our feelings and emotions. Taking a day at the spa or going on a beautiful weekend retreat isn't always in the books (or budget), but taking time to recharge is something that is crucial for all of us to do on a regular basis.

So, I started the practice of self-care in small steps, especially through these past years with difficult seasons. If I don't look after myself first, then I am no good to anyone else either. That often feels selfish, but I've had to train myself to know that it's not. I think of many people I know who have walked this journey, especially those who are primary caregivers. When you are engulfed in that world, you are just trying to survive. The idea of placing any importance on yourself feels impossible. I still struggle with this, but I'm getting better. I would imagine the same could be said for many of us. After coming up with a plan with my therapist, I was able to come up with categories of things that I do that are about taking care of myself for my own mental health. They are not complicated things; they are easy things because easy is all I can manage.

One way I look after my mental health is by doing things that bring me joy. For some reason, soup makes me happy. My lovely children told me once that I'm "very good at liquids" (not sure what that means), but I've taken it as a badge of honor. I love the process, and I realized that soup is self-care for me. Soothing to my soul. There's a recipe, but it's not too precise, so I can just go for it and get a little creative. It's warm, yummy, and makes my family happy; and that brings me a sense of calm and purpose.

I realize making soup is pretty specific and isn't for everyone, but finding something calming to do is valuable when situations in life get stressful and hard. Other things that I'd put in this category would include gardening, doing creative projects, and driving through the country with a coffee. Small things that bring little bits of joy—we can all find them and make them part of how we care for ourselves.

I also take mental breaks. Mental breaks are needed in self-care. Many days, I drive down to Lake Ontario by myself and sit and listen to the waves. We have many beautiful beach spots in our area, and I know them all well. Or sometimes, I'll wander through my favorite bookstore. Even getting away for an hour helps. When my kids were really little and I needed some space, I would go to the dollar store and look for treasures. It was my happy place. Mental breaks are different for everyone. Find out what works—something that's easy to do. Make space for those deep-breath moments in your life.

Another way I focus on self-care is I get outside. One of the best things for my mental health is going for a walk. If I'm stressed or trying to work through something in my mind, a walk always helps me focus and get fresh perspective. Nature energizes; fresh air cleanses; and blue skies calm. Standing out in the big, wide world doesn't make me feel small; it makes me feel connected and reminds me that I'm part of a greater story. Perspective is everything some days.

I also take care of myself by finding my people. One of the best practices for self-care is to build community and relationships with those who encourage you. I try to meet up for dinner regularly with two of my dearest friends. We have busy schedules, but we make it work. I have another friend whom I know I can Facetime when I need to, no matter what I look like; and my husband and I have our best couple friends with whom we love to get together and laugh, play games, and eat yummy charcuterie spreads and fancy pies. My husband and I make sure to have date nights, too, and I plan fun outings and quality time with my grown-up kids. Connecting with others in a life-giving way is an important part of self-care.

Another way to focus on my mental health is to lean into my faith. Drawing from your spiritual life can make all the difference. Sometimes, I listen to a podcast; other times, I write in my prayer journal. I can't take care of myself if I don't take care of my relationship with God. Self-care is definitely rooted in faith for me, and when I find I'm at my lowest, it's usually because I've let this slide. I can't take care of my physical and emotional self if I don't invest in my spiritual life.

We can't do all of these things all of the time. Some work better in different seasons and stages of life, and we all have our own ways to care for ourselves. Sometimes, self-care means getting professional help and talking to someone who can give you the guidance you need. If that's where you are, getting that support is the best way to care for yourself. I started seeing a therapist when my mom began to decline more rapidly because I knew I needed help coping with loss and I didn't want to find myself in a crisis down the road. Reaching out to someone is okay; we aren't meant to do life alone. Make sure that if you need extra support, you find it. There is no shame.

I've realized that I'm at my best when I remember that it's okay for me to care about me. It often feels selfish, but the better I am at looking after myself, the better I am for the people in my life whom I love.

It's a whole other story when you are a primary caregiver. I won't write the entire story of my dad in this chapter; but watching him with my mom and the way he has diligently cared for her, I definitely saw him come to the place where he needed help and time for himself, likely more than he would have ever admitted. While my visits to see my mom were, of course, for her, they were also for him. I'd send him out to the store or for a walk so that he could get some space and take those much-needed deep breaths.

When you are on the longest goodbye journey, if you are a caregiver, there will be a time when you need support—not just for basic care but also for mental health. I think, at times, it was hard for my dad to take that time for himself because it would come wrapped up in guilt. It's hard to go out and do things for yourself when the one you love can't. And often, you don't want to do anything without them. But it's so important. Even if it's just little moments. Don't feel guilty for filling your tank. Whatever your role, take the time you need and remind yourself of the value that you have, too.

Self-care is not just about spas or lavish vacations, as nice as those outlets could be. In the longest goodbye journey, self-care is the daily key to survival. It's little glimpses of light and hope in long days. It's the fuel needed to face every challenging day. Whatever you need to do, make sure to do it. Don't be afraid to care for yourself.

Reflection:

On this journey, taking care of yourself is so important. If you are a full-time caregiver, don't be afraid to ask for help or get support in place so that you can rest. Most communities have organizations that are there to help you; take advantages of those services—even if it feels uncomfortable. If you support a caregiver, it's okay to take a step back, breathe deeply, and process the season. Don't feel weak or inadequate if you need to put things in place for your own mental or physical health. Everyone needs space; boundaries are okay when you need them, and you can care for others more when you look after yourself first.

CHAPTER 10

All the Hard Things

I REMEMBER A TIME WHEN my daughter had a week that was filled with challenging experiences. Since she and I are very similar when it comes to new things, I could understand the angst and fear she was facing. In the middle of the stress she felt and trying to manage all the emotions of figuring out how to make things happen, she very loudly exclaimed, "Why do all the hard things happen at once?"

I had to think about it for a minute. It was a very true observation and a pretty good question. I've wondered that myself at times—why do we have to be brave all at once? Why does courage require every little bit of strength that we have, often in our weakest moments?

I looked at her and said what I always say, "You can do hard things."

I've said this so many times to myself over the years. I'm not sure it's my mantra, but it comes pretty close. I say it to my family when we feel challenges and have to do things that are difficult; to myself when I'm sitting alone crying in a parking lot, wondering how to process the days I'm facing; to those around me whom I see needing encouragement and hope in the stories they are living. The scale of hard things in life varies from day to day. One moment, it could be facing your first driving lesson; another day, you come face to face with something that could change the trajectory of your life. But we keep going. Amid the darkness and fear that we often face, we can have hope. Why? We *can* do hard things. I know this because I see people all around me living out their own bravery every day.

- The one facing a cancer diagnosis
- The parent believing in a healthy report for their child
- The couple trying to make their marriage work
- The parent fighting for their family
- The individual seeking direction and purpose
- The one feeling the darkness of depression
- The family watching a loved one slip away
- The person feeling a grief so strong, it hurts

As I write this chapter, we are year two into a global pandemic. If there's ever been a time when the whole world has had to both hold their breath and learn to exhale, it's now. There are hard things everywhere we look, and I see people doing all they can to overcome those hard things and press on. We are often more capable than we ever realize. Don't give up; don't despair. If you find yourself trapped by fear, wondering how you are ever going to make it out of a challenging season and be free from what hinders, you can have hope.

You don't have to be weary. *He gives strength, this anchor to the soul.*

You can stand secure. *He is steadfast and true.*

You can trust. *He is unchanging, full of grace and life.*

Keep moving forward; keep being brave. Look the situations that stare at you right in the face and remind yourself that you can do all things. You have been given all strength.

I think about walking through this season of long-term illness. Each step of this longest goodbye journey has come with its own level of grief. Everything has felt like a hard thing. There is nothing easy about losing someone you love. There is nothing enjoyable about seeing your family hurt. There is nothing about pain or loss that makes people happy.

Each stage has felt like the hardest. But we keep going. We can do hard things. I get through them because of the love I've been given and want to give. I refuse to let grief and pain steal the hope and joy that's always been present in my life. I won't let this hard thing win. It will beat me down, and it will cause me pain. But just like I told my sweet daughter in her own seasons of challenge, we can do it. And most often, we don't have a choice. I've faced doubt and insecurity at every stage of my life. And my mom was always there, cheering me on, giving me encouragement, and offering me prayers, telling me that I could do the hard things, too. So, I choose to be brave—for her and for myself. Where love is strong, loss feels deep. That's the irony of it all—the glorious mess of joy and sorrow that comes from being loved and loving in return—joy because of what you've been given, and sorrow because it doesn't last forever.

I know there are more hard days ahead, too. They won't end in this longest goodbye journey and other paths that I will have to take as I live life. But it's okay. I can do it. We can. You are stronger than you know. He is stronger than you could ever comprehend. You can do hard things because you don't have to do them alone.

Reflection:

Hard things can overwhelm us. We want to hide away under the covers and hope that everything goes away. Sometimes, when these seasons feel too much to bear, breaking all the big things down into smaller thoughts or tasks can help. The big picture of grief and loss and goodbye is overwhelming, so take each day and stage as it comes and do the best you can right there. You'll get stronger as you go. And while things will never be easy, you will learn to navigate with strength and grace as you go.

CHAPTER 11

One More Gift

I REMEMBER THE YEAR WHEN I was finally the same shoe size as my mom. I was likely around fourteen, and it seemed like I had waited years to catch up to her size eight. First, I wanted to be more like her, but the anticipation of having my shoe wardrobe double was also a very big deal. When I finally made size eight, I felt like I had arrived. From then on, my sweet mom would always share her shoes.

It didn't stop there. She actually shared everything she had with me. Always. She would give me the clothes off her back, or pulled out from her closet, or something from a shopping bag she had just bought for herself. Treasures from the cupboards, storage, boxes, and totes—almost anything you could imagine.

"You can have this," she would say.

It was just one of the million ways she would show her love to me, and since gifts are one of my love languages, my heart would be filled. Now, love expressed in this time of life is different. Sometimes, it's the recognition in her face or the slip of my name when I least expect it. Holding hands walking through the house or a cuddle together watching a movie. I treasure all these moments. But I miss sharing things with my mom. I miss her gifts—her bringing me a bag from the store or seeing me look at something in the mall and saying, "Let me get that for you." I would pretend to be surprised, but all along, I hoped she would offer. (My children have mastered this technique!) It was never because I care about things, but I knew it meant she was thinking about me. It was one of the ways she showed love to me and to all of the family. Sometimes, I think to myself, *I wish I could have one more gift* because presents remind me of presence.

One evening after my weekly supper visit to my parent's house, my dad told me to look in the front closet because there were things there that mom wasn't using anymore. It was like the make-up purge, but now, we had moved to footwear and coats. I still didn't like to take any of her belongings, but I went to look. As I peered in the closet, there was a pair of boots. Beautiful, lovely, long, black boots that she wouldn't be wearing anymore. And of course, just that week, I had said I needed new boots. As per the story of my footwear life, mine were falling apart. I hesitated as I held them in my hands.

"Take them," my dad said.

"I feel bad."

"She won't wear them again," he replied.

So, I took them.

When I got home later and put them in my closet, I remembered back to the longing of my heart—one more gift. There it was. My mama's boots. I wore them every day for the rest of the winter. And maybe it sounds silly, but I felt close to her when I put them on. I know she would have been happy that my feet were warm in all the snow; I've never been known for practical winter footwear. She would have liked them with my checkered leggings and my cute Christmas dress. I felt like her when I wore them; she's always been so stylish and beautiful, and any part of her that I can have makes me feel that way, too.

Then, as I normally do, I looked deeper and realized those boots represented other things in my life—how I'm taking giant steps of bravery every week into great unknowns and making decisions and trying to navigate middle-aged life and all that comes down the pipes. Every day is made up of a million little steps, and most of the time, they feel scary and uncertain. But

I keep walking ahead. I have my boots. I have all that my mom has given me. I don't have to be afraid of the path ahead because she's right there walking with me. Each step I take, every snowbank I trudge through, her presence is in my life. I can walk in the confidence she gave me. Literally, in her boots. Symbolically, in my life.

I've received some other gifts on this journey with her. For years, my parents would spend winter in their Florida home, and we would go and spend time with them on various occasions. A couple years ago, before my dad had to make the hard decision to sell their place because of my mom's health, my son and I made a trip down together on his spring break from university. He's always had a close relationship with his grandparents, being the first grandchild in our family, and they have a close bond. I was happy to have some time with him, and it was special for us to be there together with them. My mom was struggling then; but we took walks, went out to eat, visited Target as much as we could, and spent time together. It was our last time there with them—and likely, my last trip alone with my son, too—the now familiar mixing of joy and pain as we made memories, knowing how much things had changed. That trip was another gift I won't forget.

Another "presence present" came in the form of Facebook messages. Before my mom became sick, she was starting to use social media. I had forgotten all about it because she had stopped using it so long ago; but one night, it came to my mind, so I went back and opened my Messenger app. I spent the next couple hours crying my eyes out as I went through all the messages she had sent me over the past couple years while she still could. It was like sitting down with her, pre-Alzheimer's, and feeling the love of her words wash all over me. I could hear her voice and her heart coming through each message.

> *Keep looking up; something will come. Trust in the Lord with all your heart and lean not unto your own understanding. In all your ways, acknowledge Him, and He shall direct your paths. Love you, Mom!*

I heard Hannah's song. She did amazing; I loved it. Her singing and the song. Love you, Mom.

I love you, too, Shelly. I was soooo happy to have you here yesterday.

I really miss you a whole lot, but I understand it is important to be close to work for you and Tav, too, and I love where you are living, and I love your new home and I LOVE YOU!

The kids will be fine; they are brave. Love you, Mom.

The joy of the Lord is your strength. He equips those He calls!!!! It is always good to be nervous, and then you will totally depend on HIM. Love you . . .

Ok, now I have tears in my eyes after reading your blogs. You are sooooo special to me, Shelly, and loved dearly.

Glad you are having fun; wear your sunscreen.

I love Noah's new haircut.

Hi, Shelly. I am really missing you today. Need a mom and daughter time together. Love, Mom.

Hope you are having a great day. I am so thankful to have a wonderful daughter. You truly are the best.

Hi, Shelly. Praying that God will bless you today with favor and His wonderful blessings. You are loved dearly.

Hi, Shelly, wish you were closer. Thinking of you lots; it was such a beautiful day Saturday. Love it.

Yes, I will make you some tea biscuits.

That message is amazing. Touched a lot of hearts, including mine.

Hi, my dearest daughter. Just read your library story, I love it and can sure understand now while all these years you have grown so much into reading. And now, you have written a book, and I am sure you will have many more.

May God bless you and sustain you and pour His spirit out on you. Love you, Shelly.

And then, the last words she ever wrote to me:

I have had a good week. Love you, Shelly.

I cry every time I read through those messages. She's with me always. Her presence is strong in my life. There are many gifts to be found. I have boots. I have words. I have her silver-covered cake tray; vintage flour sifter; and the red, old-fashioned, French fry slicer. So many things that remind me of her. Presents and presence. The little girl who couldn't wait to catch up and wear her sweet mama's shoes—well, I'm the grown up now, and hopefully, the steps I take are ones worth following.

Thank you, Mama, for the boots. One more gift to add to all the gifts you have given me.

Reflection:

Gather up your gifts, whatever they may be. Words, texts, Facebook messages, old empty bottles of perfume, or even old worn boots—things don't matter, but they can bring comfort in ways that we often can't even explain. There's no right or wrong way to walk a grief journey; all is fair game when you're wrestling with loss. So, hold on to what brings you joy, make pretty boxes and fill them with precious things. Make lists, take photos, plant flowers, and do whatever it takes for you to keep going. Remembering well is a gift, and it's okay to make it whatever you need for yourself.

CHAPTER 12

Rosebud Hugs

AS I WRITE THIS CHAPTER, it's spring again. Outside the room where my mom spends most of her time, her flowers are blooming. She planted the rose bushes years ago, and trust me when I say that they are stunning. Long before I ever appreciated a flower or enjoyed any part of gardening, I was a teenager who cared more about working on her suntan than helping plant flowers or pull weeds. I remember when I got married and was obsessed with sunflowers, my mom planted some seeds for me in her front garden, mixed in with the delicate rose bushes; and they took right over, mixing the country flowers with the sophisticated blooms for the whole street to see. We laughed so hard over the wonder of it all.

And now, still, all around the outside of her house are those fingerprints of her garden love. The red, white, and deep pink roses in the front garden are definitely the show-stoppers. I also love all the vines that cover the archway going to the backyard that change color with every season. There's a beautiful white hydrangea tree and a little bush of pink peonies. I love going over during the summer, seeing what is in bloom, and taking some clips and bringing them inside the house for her to enjoy.

Then, if I take a thirty-minute drive to the family cottage, I see her flower fingerprints there, too. All around the outside are more flowers that she lovingly planted and tended. More peonies, daylilies, and ferns lovingly chosen by her and my brother. Blooming at just the right time, reminders to me of her. I've taken some home and replanted them in my own garden, too, and love to think that I'm continuing to grow things that started with her.

I'm struck by the fact that all her flowers keep coming back, year after year. My dad doesn't love gardening as much. So, over time, as my mom's health declined, there hasn't been the same kind of care, though they are still beautiful, even without her special touch and green thumb. But despite the weeds and the overgrowth that sometimes builds up, everything always blooms. No matter what happens in life, everything comes back and grows with the seasons.

Recently, I was leaving their house one day after she had been through another rough stage, and we were processing another significant decline. She wasn't able to go out anymore for her walks and drives with my dad, as her mobility had now become an issue. It made my heart so sad. As I was leaving, I glanced back at the front room of their house where she sits, and I took notice of her flowers outside the windows. I stopped dead in my tracks, and my heart pounded a little. All the flowers were in full bloom, and it was as if they were calling out to me, "We are still here. We remember! We are blooming for her. We won't forget her special touch. She is part of our glorious display."

I know plants don't have feelings, and this all might sound ridiculous; but in that moment, I imagined that all her beautiful flower friends were hugging the house knowing she was inside and remembering the care and love she gave to them when she could. Now they surrounded her still, as seasons come and go, standing on guard, a reflection of her beauty on display, never forgotten. They were sending love back to her now with their beautiful blooms. It comforted me. I was reminded that even though seasons don't look like we think they should, good things can still grow. We can see beauty; there are blooms, and growth is still possible.

And through the weeds, through the overgrowth of this longest-goodbye season, I have definitely seen things grow. The capacity to love. The strength to do things that are hard and felt impossible. Increased faith. An ability to look for joy in challenging moments. Closeness in family. Creative ways to love and support. Compassion for those hurting and alone. Extended grace in hard moments. Letting things go that don't matter. I've learned if we sow the right seeds, good things will always grow, even if life gets tangled up for a season.

I love gardening now, too. I may even be a little obsessed, year after year, as I try to fill the dirt around our home with every good thing I can find. Digging down deep and dropping in seeds, rescuing shriveled up plants from the garden center, and watching moment by moment as things begin to grow. I'm comforted to see thing come alive, and the process of new growth from dark, cold places is something that brings peace to my soul. When you think there is no hope, often, that's when new life appears. When you think things are gone, beauty will emerge. I don't quite have my mom's green thumb, but I do the best I can; and with every bloom and growth that I see, I think about her.

At her house and at mine, there are even roses that bloom late into the fall, sometimes peeking through the first blanket of snow, when things really shouldn't be growing at all. But they are always a beautiful reminder to me that life blooms in unexpected ways, too, sometimes even in unexpected seasons, assuring me that what's invested into our lives will always keep coming back and that I need to care for, value, and be deeply thankful for all that I have been given. Every year, I wait in anticipation, and the roses always bloom again.

Reflection:

We don't generally see grief as a way for us to grow in our lives. We are usually so engulfed in making it through the days that we can't identify where we are on the journey. Be assured there is growth in the longest goodbye. You will grow in ways that you never imagined, and while growth isn't always easy, it will be deposited in your life and will come back again. You may feel weak and helpless right now, but each day that you show up to be brave and face the day is a day of growth in your life. And those roots will be deep and will come back again and give you what you need for the seasons ahead.

CHAPTER 13

My Complicated Grief

I'VE OFTEN WONDERED ON THIS goodbye journey if sudden goodbyes are easier than longest goodbyes. It seems a strange thing to think about, but that's where my mind goes sometimes. I know precious people who woke up one morning to what they thought was just another day, only to experience a sudden loss of someone whom they love with no warning, no hint that an ordinary day would turn into a day of unimaginable pain. They had no signs that everything would change, that there would be no time to say goodbye, and that all the last moments were already lived. That's a deep pain to walk through—the sudden goodbye—the finality of a loss that you didn't expect. To wake up to the hope of a sunrise and go to bed that same evening under a dark cover of grief is not an easy journey.

Then I think about the longest goodbye—the years of small losses, each stage at a time, the pain that is drawn out over the years as you watch someone you love fade away. There are many people walking that journey even beyond Alzheimer's, as sickness and disease ravage bodies and life fades away.

I've come to the conclusion that there is no scale to loss. Whether your loss is sudden or drawn out, pain is pain; and walking through grief is no simple feat, whether you are faced with it unexpectedly or it's a long-haul journey. And I'm no professional grief counselor, but I think I've learned that grief is complicated, no matter what path life takes you down.

We grew up far from our grandparents and senior family members. I never watched in real time anyone whom I loved grow older, struggle with their health, and then be part of the process and journey of saying goodbye. My grandparents lived miles and miles away, and it wasn't until just a couple years ago, sitting at the bedside of my grandma, that I really saw what it was like for someone to be at the end of their life. And by that time, I was already in the middle of my own grief journey. An adult, with grown-up kids of her own, finally seeing what goodbye looked like. I felt so unprepared.

I worked as a pastor for many years, mainly focused on children and families. I always felt uncomfortable around seniors. I didn't know how to connect and was even a little afraid. I kept my distance because I couldn't function in that space. And now, life has me in this journey, in this place. And it's become my speciality, my life-lived experience.

Often, I call it a complicated grief because it's weird to miss a person when you're with them. Every week for the last five years, I have spent time with my mom. I make the thirty-minute drive usually mid-week and then on the weekend to my parents' house. We sit, talk, and catch up; my dad gets a break; we eat dinner; I wash the dishes, and my dad goes for a walk or to the store. Then I go home. I do the same the next week. And the clock keeps ticking, and soon a year has passed, and I look back and start to measure all that has been lost. And I'd miss the mom from a year ago. Or when things started to move quickly, I missed the mom from last week.

Many times, I would leave and then cry the whole drive home, which likely wasn't safe. I missed my mom. I would spend hours sitting and holding her hand, yet my heart would feel so homesick. This is a complicated grief. It's a long, long road. She'd smile and look into my eyes. I'm familiar, but she doesn't know me. That's deep pain. *I'm your girl*, I'd tell her.

As her speech started to fade, she would say things to me that I know meant much more than the words she could get out. For a season, she'd look at me and say, "You and me." Those words were a mixture of joy and pain going deep. In those three words, I know she was trying to say, "I'm so glad we are together; I'm so happy you came to see me. I'm so appreciative that you took me out to see the flowers and that we are doing the things together that we always loved. You are my daughter, and I adore you. I am still here, and I want you to know I love you. Everything that we have always had is still here. I'm your mom, and I'm still with you. I've loved you your whole life, and I still do. Don't worry, I'm here." You and me.

In another season, her phrase was, "You're so good." She'd say it to me, my brothers, and my dad. And those three words also contained more than she could express, but we knew what it meant as she looked at us with love beaming in her dark brown eyes, as she held our hand and smiled her big, beautiful smile at us. We held her tight and took her for walks and sat with our arms entwined. I know she was trying to say, "Thanks for being here for me. Thanks for loving me still. Thanks for being kind and hugging me and making sure that I'm all right. Thanks for treating me with respect and kindness, even though the days are hard. Thanks for remembering that I'm the same mom who loved you all these years. Thank you for being my family." You're so good.

This is my complicated grief—having so much and losing it all at the same time. And the more I think about it, the more I'm grateful for a long goodbye. No grief journey is easy, sudden, or long. They each come with different types of pain and different processes to walk. But I'm grateful that in the middle of my complicated grief, I have had a chance to collect moments along the way, moments I wouldn't have gotten otherwise. On this long road, I know more than ever that how we love each other when things aren't all sunny and rosy is the toughest and rawest part of life and love. For all the times that she did everything for me, now it's my time to do what I can for her.

I love you, my momma. I'll listen to your voice through my heart and live reflecting all the good you poured into my life, and I'll keep holding your hand tight and sit by your side. While my grief feels complicated, my love for you has never been clearer. I'm grateful we've had so much time to say goodbye.

Reflection:

Grief is complicated. Love is complicated. Relationships are complicated. There are no stories that are the same, no experiences alike. We can find support and help, but no one truly knows what others are feeling or going through. That's okay. How could grief be simple? How could loss be easy? How could watching someone we love slip away not be complicated? It's okay to wrestle with the complexities. It's okay to cry. It's okay to feel. It's okay to mourn. It's okay to be angry and not understand. It's okay to be filled with joy in the same moment that you feel pain. Whatever you need to do to walk the journey, let yourself feel what you need to feel. It is a complicated grief.

CHAPTER 14

The Best Dad in the World

THIS BOOK WOULDN'T BE COMPLETE if it didn't include a chapter about my dad. He's really the hero of our family. I grew up always knowing I was loved and taken care of by him. My favorite story is when he and my mom picked me up from the hospital when I was six weeks old, the baby girl they had chosen to adopt. He told my mom when they got into the car, "Lock the doors; no one is taking her back."

As a kid, I thought my dad was invincible. He could do anything. My earliest memories are of him building me the first of many special bedrooms in the basement and going out for bike rides as he towed my siblings on a wagon behind his bike. I can picture him throwing my little brothers high up into the air when they were toddlers, while they screamed in delight and my nervous mom told him to stop before someone got hurt. He could walk on his hands anywhere in the house, even off a diving board at the neighborhood pool. He was always an active and involved father. I remember sitting in the car as a young girl and feeling so safe (which is ironic considering his driving) and loved. I just knew that my dad was there for us, and he would make sure we were okay.

He was also there for others. Recently, we tried to make a list of all the people he has helped over the years, mainly doing home renovations. Pastors, friends, churches, and even organizations have been the recipient of his generous work. I think back and wonder how he found the time to basically rebuild other people's homes with his own busy schedule. But he did. Since my husband and I have been married, my dad has installed for us a new kitchen, finished two rec rooms, built one bathroom (while sick with the stomach flu on our moving day), fixed countless toilets, executed flawless plumbing jobs, constructed us a fabulous deck, and, most recently, built a roof for our pergola. My brothers could add to that list, and that doesn't even include all the work he has done for his own home and cottage over the years.

One year, my mom wanted a gazebo in their backyard, so he just started to build it. He didn't even have plans drawn. It's still there, as beautiful as ever. That kind of work is effortless for him.

The other side of my dad is the tough, no-nonsense executive, working in human resources for years doing union negotiations and managing complex organizations, where I'm sure he wasn't always the most popular guy. He is entrepreneurial, too, and owned various franchises over the years. He's been a pilot, sheriff, justice of the peace, and other roles I can't even remember. He really has done it all.

In the middle of everything, he has loved his wife and family and is a great husband, father, and grandfather. I would say, though, that his role as a grandparent has been the most enjoyable to watch. When my son, the first grandchild, was born, I think he found a reason to come over to our house *every* day to see Noah. He'd just pop in under the guise of a muffin drop-off to make himself a presence in his grandson's life.

He did that with all the grandkids. I would call him the baby hog because his sole mission was to brainwash each child to love him the most. At one year old, they would get their special handmade box from Poppy with their name on it; at ten years old, they would get 10 ten-dollar bills in a creative way. And that's just how he has always loved them. I think he did a pretty great job; they all adore him. His soft and gentle side has shone through from the love and care he's shown from the oldest to the youngest.

Then came the yellow flowers. And things began to change for him, too. Corporate life to caregiver life. Freedom to hours of isolation. Future planning to living each day at a time.

I would never assume to write my dad's story or experience; I don't fully know his internal journey or path. I do know the years have been hard, but during all the pain in this longest goodbye journey, there is no one who has made me prouder. I can only write of what I have seen and how his journey has impacted me.

My dad takes on life wholeheartedly. When faced with the new challenge of being thrust into a caregiver role, he didn't miss a beat. For many years, he kept their normal routines and rhythms. He refused to give up or tap out. He made sure my mom was still beautifully dressed. He bought her the clothes she always loved and made sure she always looked her best. During their married life, whenever he went on a business trip, he'd always come home with a beautiful new outfit for her. He prided himself on the fact he knew her size and what looked great on her, and that never changed as her disease progressed. Over the years, he made sure to get her hair cut, even colored. And at a time when most would give up, he instead learned how to do her color himself. He knew it would have mattered to her, so it mattered to him. It was incredible, really, to see the way he has honored her, especially as time has progressed.

And he has loved her unconditionally. He made sure her seventieth birthday was celebrated; we managed to make their fiftieth wedding anniversary party happen. They kept going to their winter home and summer cottage as long as possible, and every family event was celebrated as it always had been.

It's not to say that it was always easy. I imagine that it was the most painful thing, trying to go on with life with your partner present but not fully there. I don't think our family will every truly understand what he has gone through. I can't go too deep into thinking about that because my heart might split open in pain for him and all he has had to process and face. I can say that I've never seen a truer example of love and faithfulness. That will forever be his legacy to our family.

I think about the step he designed for my mom to get into the car, the bar he installed in the bathroom for her to hold on to, the special slippers he'd buy that were easy to put on, the custom seat for the bathtub. He learned how to prepare meals so that she was well-fed and made sure she had her medications and everything and more than she could ever need. In sickness and in health—he lived those words out loud.

But in the middle of all that care, I'm sure he experienced loneliness and pain that we can't understand either—the loss of a companion with whom to communicate and share life, watching her lose the memories of their life together. The loss of his freedom. These are things you can't understand unless you walk through them.

I also think about the loss of community for him. I've had to work to let some of this go because it brings up deep hurt, and I refuse to get lost in any bitterness. But I've observed when things get hard, people don't always stay. Friends fade away—those people you thought would always be there are gone. And while that hurt me as I watched, I know that must have hurt him deeper. I've prayed for deep grace because you never know what other people are walking through either. Everyone is on their own journey, and we don't know all the stories. But it also sparked something in my soul, and I'm determined to love those around me as long and as well as I can—especially in their darkest days. Isn't that what love and friendship is? Not sitting alone, wondering if anyone cares, thinking about all the people you had who are now nowhere to be found.

As years have progressed, we all realized that while our mom needed care, our dad needed support, too. That's a whole entire journey on its own. It's not easy to get caregivers to accept and realize they need help—not because they can't do it but because they need to realize that they are valuable, too, and their care is just as important.

I think our path happened in stages. Friends would occasionally come and help, so he could get a break. Then an official Personal Support Worker came at minimal hours, increasing those hours as time went on. Then the hardest stage was when things got to crisis mode and maximum support was required. All these steps took adjustment and time. This road has been a long journey.

Then there are children of caregivers, often called the in-between generation. We struggle with guilt as we try to navigate our own lives, careers, and growing families while loving and supporting those aging around us in the best way that we can. I'd be lying if I didn't say that I've lived continually with guilt. I've done my best to be there as often as I can and to support to the best of my ability. But it's never felt like enough. No one has made me feel that way; but when you see pain and isolation in action, and the people you love are hurting, you just want to immerse yourself in it all and make everything all right again. I'd do anything for my parents, but the reality is I just can't. I think at some point, caregivers and those who love and support the caregiver must acknowledge limitations and ask for grace.

Aren't we all just doing the best we can? That old familiar statement allows me to center myself. I'm doing the best that I can. I'm loving the best that I can. I can't be all things to all people always. So, I do the best with what I have. I have parents who need me, but I also have a family that needs me. I have a job to help support our family. Commitments and relationships are important to me. I need to look after my own mental health and well-being. I can't do everything all the time, but I can be present in the moments where I choose to engage and make that time matter.

My father has cared for our mom with all the love and affection possible. He can look back with no regrets, and he can be proud of all he has done. These current days, in our current stage, it's okay to need help; it's okay not to be able to do it all. Longest goodbye journeys need long-lasting grace.

If my mom could have looked into the future and seen the way that she would have been loved and cared for by my dad, she would have loved him even more than she already did. I know she would have been so proud of all that he has managed and the way he has taken on each season. All the determination he's shown in every other area of his life has been poured into her care. And there's a reason she still knows him and responds to him. He is her whole life because of all he has given to her—from the time they first met each other at a wedding to today as he sits and patiently feeds her to make sure she has all the nourishment she needs. It's heartbreak and beauty all rolled up together.

Sometimes, I send my dad a text, and I tell him he's the best dad in the world. Because he is.

Reflection:

Supporting caregivers is as important as supporting the one you are losing. Until you are in the middle of a longest goodbye journey, you can't really understand all the facets and pieces involved. You need to love but not control. Support but not take over. Guide but not demand. You have to walk another completely different journey of loss and support, usually with the one feeling the loss the most. There's no easy advice or path. Just be present. Show up. Don't disappear when things are hard. Don't stop calling because it's uncomfortable. Love the caregiver through all their grief seasons, too. They need you more than you know; don't leave them to walk the goodbye season alone.

CHAPTER 15

Legacy Love

ONE OF MY FAVORITE AUTHORS is Morgan Harper Nichols. Like most of the world, I discovered her on Instagram, noting her beautiful illustrations and poetic words. I think of her as a word artist because the way she both visually displays her thoughts along with her art is so inspiring to me. Not long ago, she had a stunning series on Instagram called, "Lessons from Monarch Butterfly Migration." It was so compelling to me to read about how it takes multiple generations of butterflies to migrate in one season. Some butterflies that begin the migration season don't make it to reach the final destination. They go so far; then others have to take over.

I hadn't heard this before, and her words and illustrations reminded me that we are all just part of a journey that continues, even after our time on earth is done. We are all part of a bigger story; we all have our part to play. It's all about legacy.

Legacy has been something that I have learned to value in my adult life. I had this revelation one day that legacy is really what you choose to make it. Even if you are in the middle of the darkest story, with the most challenging circumstances, and life seems like it has dealt you everything that could possibly work against you, you can still make the choice to change your legacy. You don't have to become your worst circumstances. I know my story and the words I write paint a picture of a healthy and happy family life, and I can acknowledge that I have been blessed when it comes to my family.

I know that not everyone would be able to or would even desire to write out the story of their family. But I believe that there is redemption in pain. There is grace for the hard things we experience. We can learn to forgive. And no matter the past, we are in control of our legacy as we move forward.

Sometimes when I get really deep in thought, I think about the generations surrounding me—families, children, grandchildren, the long line of my biological and adopted family tree—and how each generation has influenced those coming behind them, those they didn't even know. I think about what my parents have instilled into me and then into their grandchildren. I wonder what my kids will carry on from me, and I remember with a little sadness that one day I, too, will be only a memory. But I pray that I've left fingerprints on the lives around me, even though like the butterfly, I'll never really complete the journey. But I can pass on what I've learned because we are all legacy builders.

I can't think about my mom without reflecting on the legacy she has left for me. Her faith would be the greatest one. She is a woman who always loved Jesus, the Bible, and serving others. She gave those things to me, part of the legacy carried down. She also loved her family without abandon. I think my brothers and I would agree that we have had the sweetest and kindest mom our whole lives. She would do anything for us; she encouraged us; and she loved us with all that she had. She was a nurse, but she gave up her career when we were young and didn't go back to school until we were all in high school. She took a refresher course after all those years, and then she went back to work in the hospital. She then went on to help teach at the local college. She showed me what it means to be a successful working mother. She did shift work, but she still managed to be there for us. She loved my dad, and he adored her. They had a strong marriage filled with love their whole lives. They would travel, spend time with friends, and had such a full life before she got sick. They would do anything for each other—an example of marriage to me that I still hold to tightly.

Then came the grandchildren. I knew our parents loved us, but I feel like we definitely took a backseat when all the grandkids came along. My mom adored them all. Mine were the oldest, and I feel guilty sometimes that they got the best of her. They had her the longest and when she was the healthiest. But she loved each one. Her treasure, angel, princess, sunshine, jewel, star, and prince. My heart breaks a little that so many of their memories of her are when she wasn't well and when she was forgetting. But I don't want them to ever forget that she *knew* them. I watched her anticipate, celebrate, and rejoice as each one of them were born. I got the phone calls with all her stories of the grandkids. She'd tell me that she got them a stocking for their first Christmas, and she was so excited to make each one a name-card for big family dinners as our family grew. I'd go to the mall with her each time a grandchild was born, and she would get the next charm with their name for her grandma's angel's ornament. Sweet Easton was the last and the youngest, and her memory was fading; but I was with her when she got him a charm, making sure he was there, too. They were *all* deeply loved by Grandma.

And even in the end, when it likely felt scary and they didn't really know if she knew them, she knew their presence. She felt their love, and her eyes would light up whenever they were around. I know she was comforted by us all being together. Sitting around the campfire, playing the name game, watching the kids collect Easter eggs in the yard, sitting in the middle of all of the grandkids as they opened their Christmas gifts, and watching everyone throwing wrapping paper balls all around the basement, she knew love was there because the presence of family is strong.

I wish that Mom was still flying like those butterflies on that journey that Morgan Harper Nichols shared about so well. But the reality of life is that we are all just a part of that bigger picture. So, we love the best we can; we take what we learn; and we impart into the ones we love. We live with legacy-purpose because none of us really know when our time on earth will end. We don't know when our journey here will be done and we move into eternity.

All of us make many decisions each day. We react to different situations and face challenging circumstances. We walk through seasons of joy and seasons of pain. We can't control what happens in life, but we can control our part of the journey and, ultimately, what we leave behind. So, live with legacy in mind. I draw from the one I've seen and try to make choices so the one that I leave will be a beautiful reflection someday for those who come behind. I won't be the butterfly that sees the end of the journey, but I'm grateful to be part of the path.

Reflection:

Passing down a legacy is one of the greatest gifts. When you are saying goodbye to someone you love, take time to honor who they are and all that they have meant in your life. Speak of them to others; share what they meant to you. Don't let them be forgotten. Keep their memory alive, even while they are still with you. Honor and give them that dignity. When people are suffering, we often don't know how to act, so we just do or say nothing. Forgetting can feel easier. There are care homes filled with people who aren't remembered. Don't let your loved one be forgotten. If your journey with them has been hard, forgive so that your legacy can be better. Our legacy is our chance to affect the future, no matter the past.

CHAPTER 16

The Tightrope

IT'S HARD WHEN WRITING A book like this to know when to stop. Alzheimer's is an evolving disease. Just as you can't pinpoint the exact date that it began, it's difficult to keep up with the ever-moving progression of the journey. As I write these last chapters of the book, our longest goodbye story continues to evolve in real time, sometimes with no change for a month and then, suddenly, ten changes in one week.

I wrote some of these chapters years ago, and some are just a few months old. I feel as though I could keep writing forever and never know where to stop. I don't know how to measure time anymore. It's like a stopwatch that hasn't paused for the last ten years. All measured by moments. I know even by the time these words get to you that there will be many other changes, too, and our story will continue to look different.

No matter how things are measured, I won't ever forget the hardest day of my life so far. It should have been a wonderful day of celebration. But like most parts of life, joy and grief collided again into the beautiful messiness of life. This past year was a milestone year for my husband and me. A big anniversary. Because of the pandemic, we couldn't take the big trip we always dreamed of, but maybe that all worked out for the best, anyway.

There was another hard thing to face, a day when it felt almost impossible to tell myself that I could do the hard things. On the day that my husband and I were celebrating our twenty-fifth anniversary, instead of our planned weekend away, my dad, my brothers, and I were bringing my mom to her new home. Twenty-five years ago to the day, she had stood by my side at my wedding, and now, I needed to be there for her.

As I write this, it's been almost nine months since that day we moved Mom into a long-term care facility. And the longest goodbye journey is in a whole new phase now. I know that it was the right time and the best decision. She required care three times a day for just the simplest tasks, and it had become increasingly difficult for even the personal support workers (who are heroes) to manage her at-home care. But my heart still hurts if I think about it too much. I've never felt as much internal pain in the days before we all prepared for her to go. My dad received the call from the care association that there was a space available for her, and we didn't have much time to think about it all. And maybe that was for the best.

We got all the family together for one last gathering. This time, we knew it was going to be the last time—our final Easter in my parents' home together with the whole family. My daughter and I went early and set the table. I have hosted Easter at our house for the last twenty years, but this year, it had to be different, another tradition changed. So, we tried to make it as normal as we could. Easter grass explosion, little chocolate bunny trinkets on the table, and our big Easter egg hunt—all the things that I did each year that I had learned from my mom. One last time, we all gathered together back at our family home—three generations of our family.

I could barely hold it together as I thought back to all the memories we'd had with our family in that house. The teenage years. The dating seasons. Family birthdays, holidays, and countless celebrations. All our weddings. And then, the most treasured visits and sleepovers with all the grandkids. As each one of her precious family hugged her goodbye, I knew it was the ending of a beautiful era. We had held on as long as we could, and now it was time to let go. Our pain was wrapped up in all the beautiful moments we'd experienced together in that home. Our mom had loved and lived all those moments with us, and each one had meant the world to her. It hurt at the time, but when I look back, I'm so grateful that we got to all say our goodbyes there in the place where she loved us all so well.

The next morning started the hardest day I've ever experienced. My brothers, my dad, and I met early at my parents' house, so we could take her to the home together. The mom who loved us and cared for us all our lives needed us now. So, we helped my dad with packing up her things, and the five of us walked through the front door together one last time. Her house, which held all the beautiful memories and moments she loved and everything she had done over the years to make it a home, was now left behind. We brought just the essentials that she would need, her life belongings now contained in a couple plastic totes.

In my circle of friends, family, and people I follow and read, I've never heard anyone share what it's like to have to bring a family member to a long-term care facility. I'm sure there are resources out there, but I've just never come across anyone sharing what it feels like to the heart. I have to imagine there are people each day in the longest goodbye journey saying the hardest goodbyes of their lifetime and walking through it all alone.

I wish someone had warned me. I wish I knew how hard it would be. I wish that we talked about this stage of life more—when you're trying to launch your children, just coming into your own and feeling confident about your life and who you are, then having to care and support those in your life who are older and can't manage on their own. It's a complex time. Your parents have done it all for you your whole life, so now it's time for you to love and serve them. I know it's the circle of life, but we're usually too busy living it to figure it out before it happens. It's the best time of your life, mixed into the hardest moments imaginable. Days of joy, mixed in with deep grief. I wish I knew. It wouldn't make those days easier, but maybe I would have been better prepared. Or perhaps it was better that I didn't know. Maybe we'd be afraid to love with all we have if we realized that often, pain comes because of that love.

I remember when we came back from our honeymoon and stopped by my parent's house to pick up a few last things. As my new husband loaded up the car, I stood on the steps in the garage with my mom, like I had a thousand times. But this time was different; I was leaving for good. It was the last time that I would live in that house with her. After our lifetime together, from the time she brought me home in those cuddly, pink blankets, I had always been with them. I was moving only a couple blocks away to an apartment, but we both knew that everything was changing. We just held each other and sobbed on that step as we said goodbye. Life wouldn't be the same, and we both knew it.

Now this time, she was going away; it was her turn to leave. And like she had held on to me that day twenty-five years ago, it was my turn to try and hold on to her forever—a new milestone I didn't want to celebrate. But we had to let her go.

It's still fresh in my heart—the trauma of hugging her in the doorway of her new home, as strangers wheeled her away. The world was shut down because of Covid, so we couldn't even go in with her. I wanted to scream out, "That's *my* mom! You don't know her; she belongs to us. She's the most beautiful person in the world. You'd better take care of her. She's gentle and kind. She likes to be warm. She loves her tea. Put a scarf around her neck. Make sure she's okay . . . " I hugged my brothers and sobbed and sobbed that day, and many days since.

I'm grateful I can go see her now. I'm grateful for the care she is receiving. But I hate to leave her there. My dad and I both wait until her eyes close before we whisper goodbye. We don't want her to see us walk away, but eventually, we have to go. Each time, as I drive out of the parking lot, I whisper, "Bye, Mama" as I drive by her window, and I cry all the way home.

These have been the hardest of days for us all. For my amazing dad, especially. I'm so glad he doesn't have to struggle anymore, that he can rest and know she is cared for. That he's not at risk of hurting himself or burning out. But I know he grieves, too, especially that day as he went home alone—and all the days since. The pain of great love is when you have to let go. I know we still have her, and she's here with us. I'm so grateful for that. But she's not at home anymore, and I want her back. Some days, I want everything back.

Often, I close my eyes, and I'm standing on a thin and shaky wire. With one wrong lean or step either way, I might come tumbling down. I remember being a little girl at the circus, under the big top tent, watching the tightrope walker put on a show. I hold my breath and shovel popcorn into my mouth with my sticky cotton-candy hands, unable to look away as she walks across the skinny, bouncy rope in her battered and dusty ballerina-like shoes. There is tension in the air as she takes each step. Would she do it? Can she make it across?

In that case, she did. The small-town crowd cheered, and we all marveled at her skills. Ironically, as the most unbalanced, least-flexible, stunt-like person around, I relate to tightrope walkers everywhere. While I'm not suspended one hundred feet in the air (thank goodness because I'm afraid of heights), the balancing act for me most days is this continual space between joy and grief. I think I live there now; it's pretty much my home. And I try not to fall off in the middle. Happy and sad. Past and the future. The joys of life, mixed with all the hard things. In the middle of all that life has brought with my mom, I'm living those happy days, too.

Our son is getting married soon. Recently, we had a family celebration for him and his beautiful fiancée. He is the first of the next generation in our family to get married—our firstborn, the oldest grandchild in the beloved line of cousins—soon starting a life of his own. My heart was so happy. I held back tears as I snapped some pictures, remembering all the friends and family at different stages of his life. Another milestone in the journey of letting go. From little boy to soon-to-be husband.

The celebration was wonderful. I was filled with joy; laughs rang out; memories were shared; and there were smiles all around. In the middle of it all, though, I was walking that thin and shaky wire. Like the tightrope artist trying to make her way across to the other side, I was walking the line between joy and grief. With every hug, smile, and congratulations, I missed my mom, and I wanted her there. She would have been all over that day. She was with us when Noah came into the world and took his first breath, and she had never stopped caring for him or loving him as long as she could express herself.

In all the celebrations we have had lately, I imagine her there with her big smile. "Grandma's treasure is getting married," is what she would say. Instead, she was at her new home, a celebration happening that she didn't even know about.

My heart can't process that she won't be at his wedding. I can't have her beside me, beaming in pride. I want her to help me with my dreaded dress-shopping and tell me how to wear my hair. I want her in the pictures; I want to see her with all her family gathered around. In the middle of my immense joy, I feel this deep grief. But I just keep on balancing and making my way across that shaky rope.

Here's the thing about longest goodbye journeys—and perhaps most paths that we walk in life. If every day was filled with only sunshine and roses, it wouldn't be very realistic living. And if we only dealt with sadness and pain, we'd never be able to get up and face another day. The middle. The tightrope. The balancing.

By grace, that's the space where we often must live. And it's often the place where we learn to grow. Ecclesiastes 3:1-8 reminds us that there is a season for everything under the sun, and how we walk each season is significant. I don't like it, but I'm learning to embrace it. I'm navigating how to draw from both so I can keep my balance and find the moments of value in the center of it all.

I went to visit my sweet mama after the wedding shower, after our day of celebration. More than ever, I'm keenly aware of the pictures of family behind her on the wall in her new home, showing how life is moving forward. It's like a slow-motion picture, blurring around her. It moves; more photos are added as life keeps happening; but she stays still.

But she's here, and that is enough for my heart. So, I held her hand, and I told her through my tears and soaked mask all about the shower and her beautiful grown-up grandkids and the people she loves and who love her. She's happy and smiley as I talk, and I see that as another love gift from God. I feel seen and loved by her and by Him.

When I got married, sunflowers were my obsession. Before I went to see her, I bought a big bouquet of them and put them in her room on her windowsill. I held them right up to her face, and she smiled her big smile.

This memory of my wedding and our moments together connected me back to her as my son gets married. And all felt okay again. I haven't fallen off the wire. Working on my balance, even through the shaky days, I'm trying to keep in the steady center. Gathering up the joy in the moments.

Reflection:

It's not what we want to do, but we have to prepare ourselves for hard days. No matter the disease or condition, when someone we love is progressing on their goodbye journey, there is pain all along the way. We can't avoid it and pretend it's not happening, and we can't let ourselves get engulfed by it, or we'd never get out of bed again. We have to learn to walk this middle ground and love the best we can, while preparing ourselves for the next stages of pain and loss. Look for joy; it can be found even in the hardest of days.

CHAPTER 17

We Have This Hope

IT WOULD BE WRONG FOR me to assume that everyone's experience is like mine. It would be foolish to think that the love I have lived with in my family is common. I know many have walked fulfilling and life-giving paths when it comes to family. I also know that many have not. For some, the word *family* is triggering. It doesn't bring up happy emotions or great memories. For many, family is the source of pain, betrayal, and more hurt than I could ever imagine. I'm sorry if that has been your experience. While parts of my story do contain pain and hurt that I continue to work through and still manage, I know that what I have had is a gift. I also recognize that Alzheimer's affects people differently. Our experience has been hard for us, but I know hearing stories from others, that we have been blessed with how our mother has peacefully transitioned from stage to stage. Others have had to navigate symptoms and aggressions that we are grateful have not been part of our story. Regardless of our experiences, though, the path to goodbye is not easy for any of us.

But I can't help but think about second chances in longest goodbye journeys—about redemption and forgiveness. I walk through a long-term care home each week filled with people who can't care for themselves anymore, and many are alone. I wonder about their stories as they watch my dad come and visit my mom faithfully each day, or when my brothers or I come and take her for walks and give her dinner, or when the grandkids come to see her. What do the alone think? Were they loved? Did they give love? Why does no one come for them?

I believe in the hardest of journeys, it's never too late to make things right, to change the narrative, to adjust the legacy, and to find hope.

No matter what each day brings, and no matter how hard the journey feels, we can hold on tight. The sea tosses and turns; the waves roll and crash; and the ocean seems too big for us to manage on our own. And often, we can feel so small and lost in our waves of despair. Just when it's all coming down, when we're overcome and about to let go into the deep, Something steadies. Something pulls. The shoreline begins to fade from sight and feels like we are moving farther and farther away. But we are held. We don't go under because there's this Anchor that holds us secure. Hope.

In times of pain, I have hope. In times of joy, I have hope. In times of mourning, I have hope. In times of doubt, I have hope. In times of loneliness, I have hope. In times of confusion, I have hope. In times of celebration, I have hope. Jesus is the Hope Who anchors the soul.

You can find hope, too. No matter where you are in your goodbye journey, jump right into the glorious mess. Love with all you have, and don't hold back. Your anchor may be different than mine, and that's okay. But keep looking for hope even when you feel like your heart may break.

I never wanted to walk this goodbye journey. I never would have chosen to lose my mom in such a slow and painful way. I decided, though, that the love I had always received from her would be the love that I would keep giving back because she was still worthy of it all. I refused to let a lifetime of love and moments be taken from me, so instead, I went looking for all that I could hold on to.

And I have so much. From yellow flowers, boarded-up houses on the lane, butterfly journeys, stunning red roses, perfectly pink make-up, and my mama's boots, there's always been hope in the longest goodbye.

Afterword

IT'S BEEN A YEAR TO the day since we brought my mom into her long-term care home. We have lived through four seasons and navigated all the holidays and birthdays in this new normal. My amazing dad visits twice each day and helps feed her at mealtimes, then often takes her outside in her wheelchair for long walks. His care and devotion haven't changed, and I would be surprised if there's any resident who has such a consistent visitor as he. He's made friends with the staff, joined the family advisory committee, and knows many of the residents' names and stories. This year has been a huge adjustment, but I continue to be proud of him and the strength that he has shown. His unconditional love and care have continued from stage to stage, which I expected but from which I still draw inspiration.

I still make the drive from my small town twice a week for my visits. I've stopped crying when I leave, although sometimes, my eyes well up with tears as I sit beside her and share all the news. She doesn't usually respond, but I tell her all the stories of our family and show her pictures from my phone, even if her eyes are closed. Sometimes, she will smile, and I know that she feels my presence.

Her walls are papered with giant pink roses that my daughter and I hung up to surround her, and the bulletin board behind her continues to fill as we bring in new photos. I added one of my daughter's engagement pictures a few months ago and just last week the sonagram image of her first great-grandchild due later this year.

When I first started coming to visit her, I was numb, and I didn't know how to process this new environment. I would walk by all the wings labeled with house numbers and the decorative signs that said "Family," and I would stubbornly look away, not wanting to accept that this place was now where she lived and that she wouldn't be coming back to us.

But time always brings healing, and this past year I've intentionally reminded myself to keep looking for joy and hope. It's taken some time, but I finally feel at peace. I love our visits together now, and I look forward to sitting with her and especially love taking her on walks through the halls. I wave at Brenda in the room before the main door, and I stop to help sweet Jean find her way back to her room. I always smile and say hello to the two beautiful ladies who sit looking into the courtyard, one always doing a word search, and I'm captivated by the sweet couple usually sitting in the foyer watching television together. I love to watch the devoted son sitting with his father in the town square as they eat the home-cooked dinner that he brought in, and I enjoy my chats with the beautiful woman proudly wearing her gold medal from the house Olympics.

I wander through the halls, now aware of the precious people in each room. All having lived a full life, now gathered in this home, creating the most unlikely family together. Then we keep walking, down the hall lined with beautiful pink orchids that always seem to bloom, across to the hall with the bright windows that look out into a mini replica of her town with the old train station. The display cases are filled with seasonal decor and photos of the residents, and I have finally come to terms with the fact that this is, indeed, a beautiful place filled with special people living out the final years of their lives together. Home.

I'm not angry or filled with grief anymore, just incredibly thankful that I still have my mom, that she's being cared for, and that I can come and be with her. I count our moments together as joy, even in the middle of my ongoing loss.

There's a display wall that I avoided looking at for a long time; it's a memory board in the main gathering space. It lists the names of the beloved people who have passed on. At first, I couldn't look, I didn't want to know how fast the names would change, and I didn't want to think about the name of the one I love up there. But I've come to understand so much more about the dignity of life and the importance of deep love and honor at each stage. So, now I stop in a moment of respect and silence, and I look at the names and try to memorize them until the next time I walk by. A gentle reminder to me also not to take any moments I still have with my mom for granted.

And so, the seasons go on. Soon the mama duck and baby duckling will return to the courtyard just outside my mama's room, and the second year marked in her home will begin. So much has changed, maybe me the most, and I have peace as I keep finding hope in our longest goodbye. I think back some days to that last message I found on Facebook from her, and it gives me comfort. I imagine it's what she says to me each time I come and leave.

"I have had a good week. Love you, Shelly."

And I know, no matter what is ahead, I will be okay.

Acknowledgments

THANKS TO MY FAMILY FOR all their support as we've walked this journey together.

Tav, you're an amazing husband, and I'm so glad to live both my hardest days and my greatest days with you. Thanks for always telling me that it's going to be okay. I love you so much!

Noah and Hannah, I love you with all I have. You've always cheered me on in all my dreams and are the best kids a mom could ask for!

Annie and Kurtis, I'm so blessed to be your "bonus" mom. You've made our family complete.

Dad, you are my hero. I love you forever and always. I'll tell stories of you to my grandchildren about how you loved us all so well.

Blair and Kirk, I know we have each felt the loss of our mom so deeply through this journey and grieved our own ways. I love you both so much, and I know Mom would be so proud of you.

Tanja, Michelle, Kaite, Jaina, Jared, Nixon and Easton, Mom and Grandma loved you all SO much; family was everything to her. Always remember how special she thought you all were.

Thanks to the healthcare workers who are committed to caring for seniors. You are bright lights; so many of you have blessed our family over the past years, and we are so grateful.

Additional Resources

Arden, Jann. *Feeding My Mother: Comfort and Laughter in the Kitchen as My Mom Lives with Memory Loss*. Random House Canada, 2017.

Folgeman, Dan, creator. *This is Us*. Los Angeles, CA: 20th Century Fox, 2016.

Glatzer, Richard and Wash Westmoreland, dirs. *Still Alice*. Culver City, CA: Sony Picture, 2015. DVD.

Nichols, Morgan Harper (@morganharpernichols). "Lessons from Monarch Butterfly Migration." *Instagram*, May 5, 2021. https://www.instagram.com/p/COf9VcRsGtc.

For more information about

Shelly Calcagno
and
The Longest Goodbye
please visit:

www.shellycalcagno.com

Ambassador International's mission is to magnify the Lord Jesus Christ and promote His Gospel through the written word.

We believe through the publication of Christian literature, Jesus Christ and His Word will be exalted, believers will be strengthened in their walk with Him, and the lost will be directed to Jesus Christ as the only way of salvation.

For more information about
AMBASSADOR INTERNATIONAL
please visit:

www.ambassador-international.com
@AmbassadorIntl
www.facebook.com/AmbassadorIntl

Thank you for reading this book. Please consider leaving us a review on your social media, favorite retailer's website, Goodreads or Bookbub, or our website.

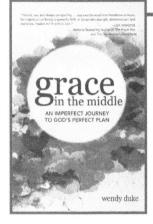

Grace in the Middle is a memoir recounting one young couple's struggle to hold on to an unraveling faith during the greatest crisis of their lives. Heartbreaking, triumphant, and funny in just the right places, this inspiring story is an authentic reflection on battling and overcoming physical illness and disability, resisting the dark doubts that plague us in the midst of tragedy, and trusting the faithfulness of God through the deep twists and turns of life.

Vanna Nguyen had escaped a war-ravaged Vietnam to make a life in America. Life seemed good and was finally settling down as Vanna planned a graduation party for her daughter Queena. But one phone call completely derailed those plans and sent Vanna and her daughters down a road that they had never dreamed they would travel. The Bloomingdale Library Attack Survivor made a name for herself, but in a way no mother would ever want. Read about two women from the same family who fought against all odds to "make beauty from ashes."

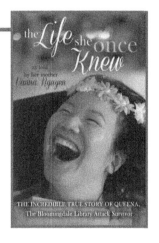

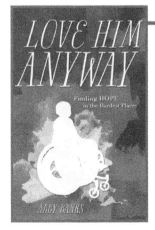

One night can change everything. Abby Banks put her healthy, happy infant son to sleep, but when she awoke the next morning, she felt as though she was living a nightmare. Her son, Wyatt, was paralyzed. In an instant, all her hopes and dreams for him were wiped away. As she struggled to come to grips with her son's devastating diagnosis and difficult rehabilitation, she found true hope in making a simple choice, a choice to love anyway—to love her son, the life she didn't plan, and the God of hope, Who is faithful even when the healing doesn't come.